CW01654224

QUIZZES AND QUESTIONS FOR NURSES

Book A. Medical Nursing and Paediatric Nursing

QUIZZES AND QUESTIONS for Nurses

Book A. Medical Nursing and Paediatric Nursing

E. J. HULL BA, SRN, RNT
Formerly Principal Tutor, Luton and Dunstable Hospital

B. J. ISAACS SRN, Part 1 CMB, RNT
Director of Nurse Education, Bedfordshire Area Health Authority; Member of the Examining Board of the General Nursing Council for England and Wales

Baillière Tindall London Philadelphia Toronto
Mexico City Rio de Janeiro Sydney Tokyo Hong Kong

Baillière Tindall 1 St Anne's Road
W. B. Saunders Eastbourne, East Sussex BN21 3UN, England

West Washington Square
Philadelphia, PA 19105, USA

1 Goldthorne Avenue
Toronto, Ontario M8Z 5T9, Canada

Apartado 26370—Cedro 512
Mexico 4, DF Mexico

Rua Evaristo da Veiga 55, 20° andar
Rio de Janeiro — RJ, Brazil

ABP Australia Ltd, 44–50 Waterloo Road
North Ryde, NSW 2113, Australia

Ichibancho Central Building, 22–1 Ichibancho
Chiyoda-ku, Tokyo 102, Japan

10/fl, Inter-Continental Plaza, 94 Granville Road
Tsim Sha Tsui East, Kowloon, Hong Kong

© 1976 Baillière Tindall

All rights reserved. No part of this publication may be reproduced, stored in a retrieval system or transmitted, in any form or by any means, electronic, mechanical, photocopying or otherwise, without the prior permission of Baillière Tindall, 1 St Anne's Road, Eastbourne, East Sussex BN21 3UN, England

ISBN 0 7020 0598 3

First published 1976
Third edition 1982
Reprinted 1985

Printed in Great Britain by Biddles Ltd, Guildford and King's Lynn

CONTENTS

PREFACE

The ideas behind *Quizzes and Questions for Nurses* are similar to those underlying our previous series, *Do-It-Yourself Revision for Nurses*. It aims to provide a plan of revision, based on examination questions and 'model answers'.

In the present books, however, the majority of the questions are taken from papers set for the assessment of pupil nurses; but, as they all deal with topics and situations met by *all* nurses, we hope that they will be helpful not only to pupils but to student nurses as well, especially in the earlier part of their training. Although the scope of knowledge is somewhat less than in the former books, we hope we have set a standard acceptable for any learner engaged in basic nurse training.

We have somewhat modified our plan in the 'revision' part of each chapter. Instead of the simple list of 'Points to revise' which we gave in our former books, the revision takes the form of a quiz, with answers and explanations, covering all the material needed for answering a question. We hope in this way to give learners more guidance in their revision.

After the revision quiz and explanations comes the question, to be answered as far as possible under examination conditions; and this is followed by a 'model answer' with a marking scheme by which the learner can mark her own work. The method of using the book is explained in more detail in the Introduction.

We hope that those who use the books will find this method interesting, helpful and encouraging.

February 1976

E. J. Hull
B. J. Isaacs

Introduction

TO THE STUDENT—HOW TO USE THIS BOOK

DO NOT SKIP THE INTRODUCTION: it shows you how to get most help from the book.

(a) You will see that there are two main sections in the book: Medical Nursing and Paediatric Nursing. The book has been written to help you to *revise*; so you should only tackle chapters in a section when you have already had the right type of experience, i.e. if you have worked on medical wards but not on paediatric ones, start with the 'Medical Nursing' section, and leave 'Paediatric Nursing' until you have been on a children's ward.

(b) Following each main section there are some 'General' Nursing questions. You may be able to answer these whatever experience you have had.

(c) Even if you have not been nursing for very long, you have had *some* experience, and should be able to answer some of the questions. So start revising in good time, and don't leave all your revision until the last weeks before your examination.

(d) Each chapter in the book starts with a lot of very short 'revision questions'—a *quiz* covering some part of the syllabus. You must answer these questions FIRST. You can do them on your own or discuss them in a group. In either case, WRITE DOWN the answers. In some of the questions you simply have to choose the right answer from several alternatives; in others you have to write a few words or draw a diagram. When you have finished this, find the correct answers on the next page. There is also some explanation of the answers. You correct your own answers and see how well you have scored. The idea is to help you to recall what you do know and show you what you don't.

NOW, do any more revision you need, and fill in gaps you have found in your knowledge.

(e) So far, so good. But in your examinations, as you know, you do not always have a quiz with very short answers, but may have to write longer answers, each taking about 40 minutes. So the second part of each chapter gives you practice in this. There is a question to be answered under examination conditions, which you should answer without looking back or using books, allowing yourself not more than 40 minutes. Needless to say, the quiz and the question do not *have* to be done on the same day.

(f) When you have written your answer (NOT before), you turn to the next page. Here there is a 'model answer', with a scheme for marking your own work. You should do this as soon as possible.

The first section contains a quiz and a question for practice, with some advice on marking.

NOW START on the quiz on the next page.

Practice Quiz and Question

1 THE LARGE INTESTINE: CONSTIPATION

REVISION QUIZ

1. Here is a diagram of the large intestine. Name the parts marked A to G.

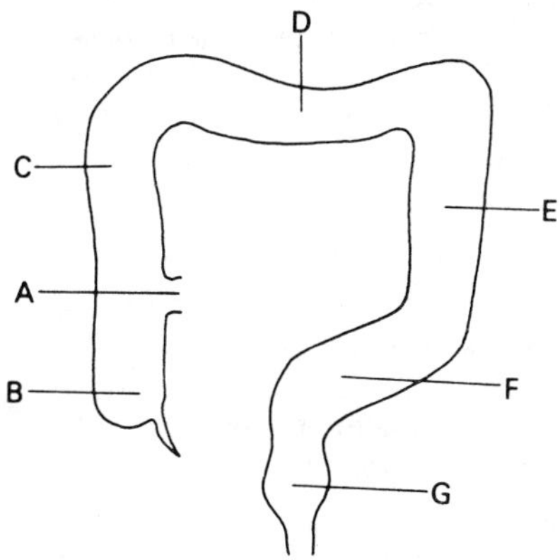

2. *Copy* the diagram and make sure you could draw it from memory.

In each of the remaining questions there is only ONE correct answer. You have to choose this, so write A, B, C, etc., ONLY.

3. Are the contents of the large intestine called

   A. chyme B. chyle
   C. faeces D. roughage

4. In the parts of the above diagram labelled B and C, are the contents

   A. liquid B. semi-solid C. solid

5. In the part labelled F are the contents

   A. liquid B. semi-solid C. solid

6. Is the part labelled G normally

   A. full B. empty most of the time

7. Are the contents of the intestine moved along

A. by gravity
B. by the muscles of the abdominal wall
C. by peristalsis
D. by the pressure of food coming from behind

8. Is the inside of the large intestine normally

A. sterile
B. full of disease-producing bacteria
C. full of bacteria which do not produce disease

9. A boy of 12 is confined to bed with a fracture of the tibia. He has not asked for a bedpan for two days. Would you

A. wait for him to ask for one
B. tell him to be sure to ask if he needs one
C. persuade him to try to use one after breakfast each day
D. ask Sister if you should give him a suppository

10. As this boy is becoming constipated, which of the following would be the more suitable breakfast for him

A. porridge, bacon, brown bread and butter and jam, with tea to drink
B. rice crispies, boiled egg, toast and marmalade, with milk to drink

11. Which of the following would be most suitable for his lunch

A. fish and chips, followed by steamed pudding
B. steamed fish and mashed potatoes, baked custard and tinned fruit
C. roast meat, baked potatoes, greens and an apple

12. Which would be most suitable for his tea

A. toasted cheese, followed by ice cream
B. sardines with lettuce and tomatoes, followed by prunes and custard
C. scrambled eggs on toast, followed by jelly and custard

Now correct your answers from the notes on pages 5 and 6.

ANSWERS AND NOTES ON REVISION QUIZ

For question 1 count ONE mark for each item correctly named.

1. A. small intestine (*or* ileocaecal valve)
   B. caecum
   C. ascending colon
   D. transverse colon
   E. descending colon
   F. sigmoid colon (*or* sigmoid flexure)
   G. rectum

Total=7 marks.

For questions 3–12 count TWO marks for each correct answer.

Correct answer

3. C. The contents of the large intestine are *faeces.* They are partly composed of roughage, the part of food which cannot be absorbed, but also contain water, bacteria and debris (refuse) from the intestines.

4. A. Faeces are liquid in the first parts of the large intestine.

5. C. As one of the main functions of the large intestine is to absorb water, faeces have become solid, by the time they reach the sigmoid colon.

6. B. The rectum is empty most of the time. It is filled by a wave of peristalsis about once every 24 hours. This produces the feeling of wanting to open the bowels.

7. C. *Peristalsis* is the movement of the muscular walls of the alimentary tract, which pushes the contents along.

8. C. The large intestine contains large numbers of bacteria, mostly non-pathogenic (*not* disease-producing) such as *Escherichia coli*. They help to form the faeces by breaking down roughage and also produce vitamins as they do this.

9. C. You should make sure that the boy has a bedpan regularly at the same time each day, after breakfast being the most usual time for the rectum to become full. He may not ask because of not liking the idea of using a bedpan, or from shyness. Make sure curtains are drawn round the bed, so that he has some privacy.

Lying in bed, change in meal times, and perhaps not having eaten much because of his accident are likely to cause constipation; so he *may* need a suppository at first; but should be encouraged to develop regular habits again.

10. A.
11. C.
12. B.

The point about these meals is that they all contain food with roughage: porridge, brown bread, vegetables, especially raw ones, and fruit.

Maximum Total = 27 marks.

Your score will show you how well you have done. Do any more revision which you think you need BEFORE attempting the question on the page opposite.

QUESTION

Without looking back or consulting any book, write the answer to the question on this page. You should not take more than 40 minutes to plan and write your answer.

A schoolboy confined to bed after a road accident is constipated.

(a) Give a short account of the large intestine and its functions.
(b) List the possible causes of this patient's constipation.
(c) How may it be relieved without the use of aperients?

READ THE QUESTION CAREFULLY. Underline words such as 'list' and 'without the use of aperients', otherwise you may waste time writing what examiners call 'irrelevant matter'.

When you have finished your answer, and not before, turn over and correct it by the 'model answer' overleaf.

MODEL ANSWER

Note on correcting answers. You will have found it quite easy to correct the *quiz*; but correcting answers to questions needs more judgement. This is because no two people will write an answer in exactly the same words, or put the different points in quite the same order. So look for the *points*, not exact words. If you have the same point in different words, count the marks for it. Examples of different ways of saying the same thing are given in brackets, thus (*or* . . .), but there will still be other ways in which you may have made the same point.

Now correct your work by this *model answer*.

(a) *The large intestine* (50 marks)

This is the last part of the alimentary (*or* digestive) tract (1). It is about 2 metres (*or* 6 feet) long (1). Count THREE marks for the correct shape of diagram and ONE mark for each part correctly labelled (= 10 marks).

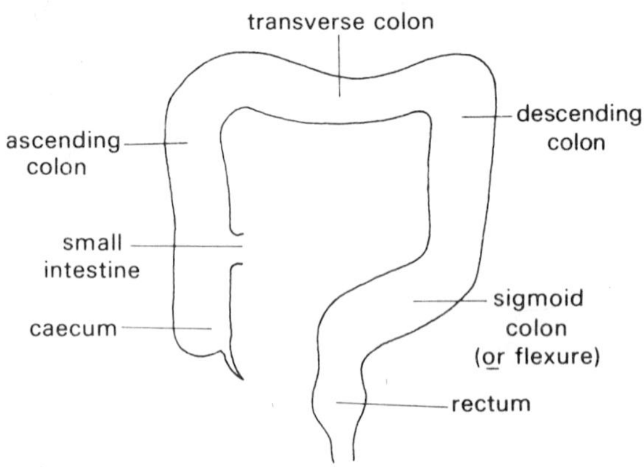

The small intestine joins the first part of the large intestine (1). The pouch called the caecum (1) leads into the ascending colon (1); the next parts are the transverse (1) and descending colon (1). The sigmoid colon (*or* flexure) (1) leads to the rectum (1), which is straight (1) and normally empty (1).

(*Note* how many words you can save by drawing a diagram. If you have no diagram you would need to describe the direction in which the different parts go, to say that the sigmoid is S-shaped, etc., and that the caecum is a blind pouch. All this is shown by a diagram.)

The contents of the intestine are called faeces (1) and consist of roughage (*or* the indigestible part of food) (2), water (2) and debris (*or* dead cells, refuse, etc.) from the intestines (2). Faeces also contain many bacteria (1).

The intestine absorbs water (4), so the faeces are liquid in the first part (2), but are solid when they reach the rectum (2). They are moved along by peristalsis (3), the movement of the muscular walls of the intestine (1). Normally a wave of peristalsis fills the rectum about once in every 24 hours (3). This leads to the feeling of wanting to open the bowels (*or* defaecate) (2).

Vitamins are made in the large intestine (3) through the action of bacteria on its contents (1).

(b) *Causes of the boy's constipation* (20 marks)

Missing meals (*or* irregular meals, change in normal routine) (4); insufficient fluid intake (4); lack of exercise (4); insufficient roughage in the diet (4); and difficulty in or dislike of using bedpans (4).

(*Note:* the question asked for a *list* of causes; so you should not have wasted time writing a lot about them. But you can count the marks for any of the above points mentioned.)

(c) *Relief of constipation* (30 marks)

The boy should be encouraged to eat well (4), and be given some extra fruit (4) and other sources of roughage such as brown bread (2), cereal containing roughage (*or* examples such as porridge, All-bran, etc.) (2) and salads (2). He should also be encouraged to drink plenty (3).

He must be encouraged to try to use a bedpan regularly (4), and must be given sufficient privacy by having curtains drawn round the bed (3). If it is possible to get him out of bed he would find it easier to use a commode (*or* Sani-chair) (3).

Suppositories may be needed at first, until his bowels have got into a regular routine again (3).

Now add up your marks. It is a good idea to keep a record of your marks for each question. You will find that they improve as you get more practice in writing answers. If you do get poor marks for a question, you will learn quite a lot as you correct your answer. You can prove this if you try the same question again after a few weeks. For a pass, you should aim at getting 55 to 60 marks out of 100 on a question. If you get 70, you are probably doing very well. In an examination, hardly anybody ever writes a *perfect* answer!

Medical Nursing

2 PEPTIC ULCER AND DIGESTION

REVISION QUIZ

In each of questions 1–7 there is only ONE correct answer. You have to choose this; so write A, B, C etc. ONLY.

1. Does a 'peptic ulcer' mean an ulcer

   A. in any part of the digestive system
   B. in the duodenum
   C. in the stomach
   D. in either the stomach or the duodenum

2. A drug used in the treatment of peptic ulcers is cimetidine. Does this drug

   A. neutralize acid in the gastric juice
   B. limit the secretion of gastric juice
   C. help the patient to rest and stop worrying

3. Are the above drugs given

   A. before meals   B. after meals

4. Antacids, such as magnesium trisilicate and aluminium hydroxide, are also used. Do these

   A. neutralize acid in the gastric juice
   B. limit the secretion of gastric juice
   C. help the patient to rest and stop worrying

5. Are antacids given

   A. before meals   B. after meals

6. Which of the following drugs is most likely to be given to a patient suffering from a peptic ulcer

   A. morphine   B. pethidine
   C. aspirin   D. diazepam

7. Ascorbic acid tablets may be given because the diet does not contain enough

A. vitamin B | B. vitamin C
C. iron | D. roughage

Now WRITE the answers to the following questions

8. Which *five* of the following foods are likely to be *omitted* from the diet of a patient suffering from peptic ulcers

A. lettuce | B. sieved cabbage | C. strawberries
D. meat | E. poached eggs | F. fried eggs
G. bramble jelly | H. chutney | I. chips
J. mashed potatoes

9. Apart from the *choice* of foods, what do you think is the most important rule about feeding a patient with a peptic ulcer?

10. Make a list, in correct order, of the parts of the digestive tract through which food passes.

11. The movement of the muscle in the walls of the digestive tract which moves food along is called (write down the missing word).

12. Make a list, in correct order, of the digestive juices which act on food.

13. Foods become soluble because of present in the digestive juices (write down the missing word).

14. List the soluble forms of

A. protein | B. carbohydrate | C. fat

which are the end products of digestion.

Now correct your answers from the notes on the pages 13 and 14.

ANSWERS AND NOTES ON REVISION QUIZ

For questions 1–7 count TWO marks for each correct answer.

Correct answer

1. D. An ulcer in either the stomach *or* the duodenum.

2. B. Belladonna and probanthine limit secretion of gastric juice.

3. A. *Before* meals.

4. A. Antacids neutralize acid in the gastric juice.

5. B. *After* meals.

6. D. Phenobarbitone (or a tranquillizer such as diazepam) is often given to help a patient to rest and not to worry, as stress is believed to be a cause of peptic ulcers. Morphine and pethidine would usually *not* be given, because they cause addiction. Potassium citrate mixture is a urinary antiseptic—no reason to give it to this patient!

7. B. Ascorbic acid is vitamin C. It is present in fruit, e.g. citrus fruit and blackcurrants, and green vegetables; the diet given to patients with peptic ulcers does not contain much of these.

For questions 8–14 count marks as shown.

8. A, C, F, H, I (1 for each = 5 marks). Foods omitted are raw vegetables and fruit (lettuce, strawberries); fried foods (fried eggs, chips), highly spiced or acid foods (chutney). *Sieved* vegetables can be given, and preserves such as jelly not containing pips and skins.

9. Small, frequent meals with milk drinks between (2). The stomach should not be left empty or acid gastric juice collects and irritates the ulcer.

10. Mouth, pharynx, oesophagus, stomach, small intestine, large intestine (*or* colon) (1 for each, but only if in correct order, =6 marks).

11. Peristalsis (2).

12. Saliva, gastric juice, bile/pancreatic juice, intestinal juice (1 for each, but only if in correct order, =5).

13. Enzymes (2).

14. Soluble form of A. (protein) is amino acids (1), of B. (carbohydrate) is glucose (1), and of C. (fat) is fatty acids and glycerol (1).

Maximum Total=39 marks.

Your score will show you how well you have done. Do any more revision which you think you need BEFORE attempting the question on the page opposite.

QUESTION

Without looking back or consulting any book, write the answer to the question on this page. You should not take more than 40 minutes to plan and write your answer.

Mr Robertson has a peptic ulcer and is in hospital.

(a) What diet and treatment may be ordered for him?
(b) Describe briefly the process of digestion.

(*Hint to the student*. Notice that in part (b), you are *not* asked to describe all the organs of the digestive system. You will not have time to do this; you only have to describe what happens to food as it passes through the organs.)

When you have finished your answer, and not before, turn over and correct it by the 'model answer' overleaf.

MODEL ANSWER

(a) *Diet and treatment* (50 marks)

Mr Robertson will need small, frequent feeds or meals (3). If he is having a great deal of pain, he may be given two-hourly (2) drinks of milk (2). This will be gradually increased so long as he is free from pain (2), by adding small quantities of easily digested foods (1), such as lightly boiled or poached eggs (1), bread and butter (1), steamed fish (1), minced meat (1), sieved vegetables (1), or anything which does not cause him pain (1). Things which will be omitted are fried foods (1), alcohol (1), highly spiced foods (1), raw fruit and vegetables (1), or anything containing a lot of roughage (1). Some milk should be available on his locker for him to drink in the night (1).

He should be encouraged not to smoke (2). He will probably need a regular aperient such as lactulose (2) because his diet does not contain enough roughage (1); and ascorbic acid tablets (2), as it may be deficient in vitamin C (1).

He may be given cimetidine tablets or carbonoxolone tablets or capsules (2 for each drug) to aid the healing of the ulcer (1). He will probably be given an antacid (2) to neutralize acid in the gastric juice (2) *after* meals (2), e.g. mist. magnesium trisilicate, aluminium hydroxide (1 for any example of an antacid you have seen given).

Rest and freedom from worry are very important (2). He may have to rest in bed for a time (2). The medical social worker should see him in case he has any worries which she can help to sort out (2). He may require a drug such as diazepam as prescribed to help him to rest (2).

(b) *Digestion* (50 marks)

In the mouth, food is broken up by the teeth (1) and moistened by saliva (1). It is swallowed, passing through the pharynx (1) into the oesophagus (1). Food is then passed down the digestive tract by peristalsis (3), which is the action of the muscular walls of the tract (2). It passes into the stomach (1), where it remains for two to four hours (2); then into the duodenum (1) and the rest of the small intestine (1). Here all the food substances are absorbed (1) through the villi (1). The residue passes into the large intestine (*or* colon) as faeces (1).

As food passes down, it is mixed with digestive juices (2): saliva (2), gastric juice (2), bile (2), pancreatic juice (2) and intestinal juice (2). These contain enzymes (3), which make the food more and more soluble as it gets further along the tract (3). In the small intestine all the food substances have become soluble (2); proteins have become amino acids (3), starch and sugar (*or* carbohydrates) have become glucose (3) and fats have become fatty acids and glycerol (3). They can then be dissolved in the water from the digestive juices (3) and are ready to be absorbed (1).

Medical Nursing

3 HAEMATEMESIS

REVISION QUIZ

In each of questions 1–5 there is only ONE correct answer. You have to choose this; so write A, B or C., etc., ONLY.

1. Is haematemesis caused by

   A. perforation of a gastric ulcer
   B. perforation of a duodenal ulcer
   C. bleeding from a gastric ulcer
   D. all three of the above

2. You are preparing for the admission of a patient who has had a severe haematemesis. Which of the following would you NOT need to have in readiness

   A. extra pillows
   B. an infusion stand
   C. a sphygmomanometer
   D. equipment for an injection
   E. a bed elevator

3. Would this patient be likely to have

   A. a high blood pressure and a rapid pulse
   B. a high blood pressure and a slow pulse
   C. a low blood pressure and a rapid pulse
   D. a low blood pressure and a slow pulse

4. Would this patient's skin feel

   A. hot and sweaty
   B. cold and sweaty
   C. hot and dry
   D. cold and dry

5. When this patient is discharged, would you tell him to

   A. avoid eating between meals
   B. have snacks between meals

Now WRITE the answers to the following questions.

6. Which FIVE of the following should the patient, convalescent after a haematemesis, be advised to avoid

A. roast lamb	B. cigarettes	C. honey
D. mint sauce	E. cold ham	F. raw apples
G. stewed apples	H. tinned peaches	I. beef steak
J. raspberry jam	K. cocktails	L. rice pudding

7. Here is a diagram of the stomach, Name the parts labelled A to G.

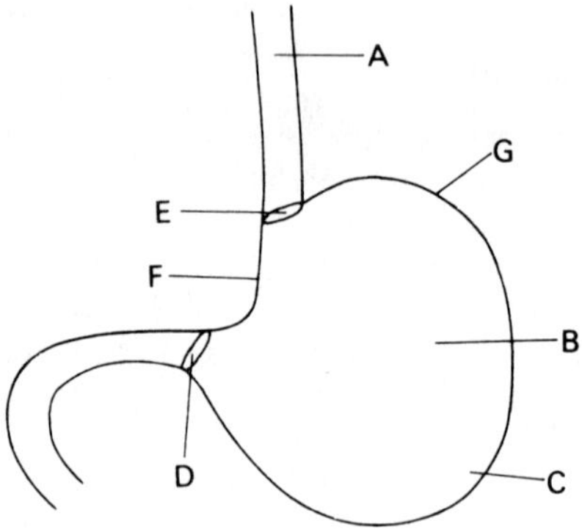

Now correct your answers from the notes on the pages 19 and 20.

ANSWERS AND NOTES ON REVISION QUIZ

In questions 1–5 count TWO marks for each correct answer.

Correct answer

1. C. In *perforation*, the ulcer 'eats through' the stomach wall and there is leakage of the stomach contents into the peritoneal cavity. There is *no* bleeding.

2. A. The patient will be shocked and therefore should not sit up as blood, and oxygen, is required by the brain.

3. C. This is a sign of shock. (If you chose the wrong answer, look up the chapter on 'Shock and haemorrhage' in any first-aid or surgery textbook.)

4. B. Another sign of shock.

5. B. The patient may feel discomfort if the stomach becomes empty; this can often be relieved by a drink of milk or a snack.

In questions 6 and 7 count ONE mark for each correct item.

6. B. Smoking is an irritant to the stomach, especially before meals.
   D. Mint sauce is made with vinegar which is very acid and may cause discomfort.
   F. Raw fruit tends to be indigestible (whereas stewed fruit, if it does not contain pips or skins, is safe).
   J. Raspberry jam is much too 'pippy'; jelly-type jams are safe.
   K. Alcohol is also a stomach irritant.

Total=5 marks.

7. A = oesophagus
   B = body (*or* cavity) of stomach
   C = greater curvature
   D = pylorus (*or* pyloric sphincter)
   E = cardiac orifice (*or* cardiac sphincter, *or* cardia)
   F = lesser curvature
   G = fundus

Total=7 marks.

Maximum Total=22 marks.

Your score will show you how well you have done. Do any further revision you think you need BEFORE attempting the question on the page opposite.

QUESTION

Without looking back or consulting any book, write the answer to the question on this page. You should not take more than 40 minutes to plan and write your answer.

A business executive aged 60 years is being admitted to a medical ward with haematemesis.

(a) What is meant by the term 'haematemesis'?
(b) What nursing care would this patient require on admission?
(c) What advice would you give to this patient about his diet before he goes home?
(d) Draw and label a simple diagram of the stomach.

When you have finished your answer and not before, turn over and correct it by the 'model answer' overleaf.

MODEL ANSWER

(a) *Haematemesis* (5 marks)

This means vomiting blood from the stomach (5).

(b) *Nursing care on admission* (55 marks)

When he is brought to the ward, the patient should be lifted (1) on to the bed and laid flat (3) with one, soft, protected pillow (2) under his head (1).

He should be moved as little as possible (2) and handled gently (1) to prevent further bleeding (1).

A vomit bowl and cloth (*or* paper wipes) should be within reach (2).

His temperature (1), pulse (1), respiration (1) and blood pressure (1) are taken and recorded. If his pulse is over 100 and his blood pressure under 100 mmHg the foot of his bed should be raised (3).

Any dentures should be taken out and cleaned (2) and placed in a labelled container (2) in a safe place (1). He can be helped to have a mouthwash (2). His hands and face can be sponged (2).

His wife may stay with him until the doctor comes (3) and she should be reassured that the patient is in good hands (2). Before leaving, she should be given the telephone number (1) and told when to enquire (*or* visit) (2).

The patient should be offered a urinal (1) and his urine tested (1); the test results should be charted (1). A fluid balance chart should be started (2). If a stool is passed, it should be saved for inspection (2). Any vomit must also be saved (2).

He may be allowed ice to suck, but nothing else should be given to eat or drink (2). The nurse can prepare an intravenous infusion trolley (2).

Pulse and blood pressure recordings are made every half hour (1) and any rise in pulse, fall in blood pressure or change in colour to ashen grey reported at once (3).

Any complaint of pain should also be reported (1).

(c) *Advice about his diet* (30 marks)

He would be advised to eat small meals (2) at frequent (*or* two-hourly) intervals (2); not to hurry over meals (2) and to chew his food well (2).

He should drink at least 0.5 litre (*or* 1 pint) of milk daily (2) and always carry milk chocolate or biscuits in his pocket (2 for either) when he goes out (1).

Food to avoid (count FIVE marks for any five): red meat (*or* beef); foods containing roughage (*or* green vegetables, salads); brown bread; raw fruit; fried foods; pastry; highly spiced foods; highly seasoned foods; alcohol; strong tea and coffee.

Foods easy to digest (count FIVE marks for any five): lean white meat (lamb, chicken, rabbit); eggs; cream cheese; milk dishes; white fish; sponge cakes; honey; jelly; ice-cream; stewed fruit; sieved vegetables; some tinned fruit (with no pips, skins).

He should not smoke (2), especially before meals.

As his ulcer heals, he can increase his diet (2); he will find out what foods cause discomfort and avoid them (3).

(d) *A simple diagram of the stomach* (10 marks)

Count THREE marks for the correct shape and ONE mark each for the labels indicated on the diagram below.

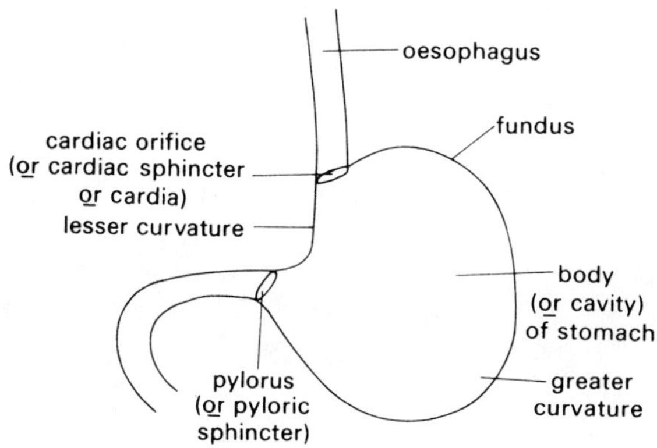

Medical Nursing

4 THE HEART AND CONGESTIVE HEART FAILURE

REVISION QUIZ

1. This diagram shows the heart and the large blood vessels which carry blood into and out of the heart. Name the parts labelled A to I.

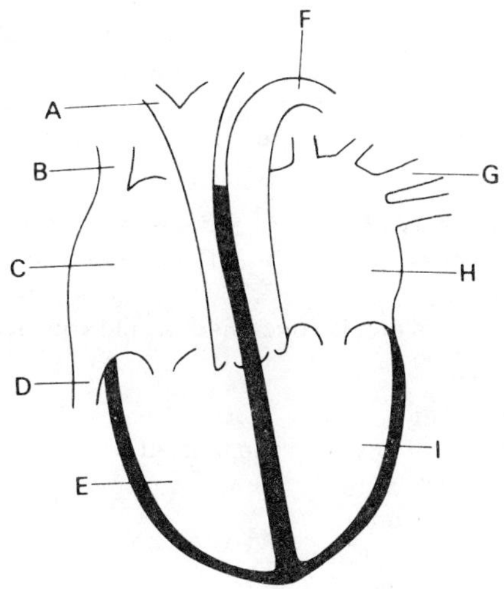

2. Which of the blood vessels shown above carry blood *into* the heart?

3. Which blood vessels carry blood *out* of the heart?

4. Which of the blood vessels carry oxygenated blood?

5. Which of them carry deoxygenated blood?

6. A patient is to be admitted to the ward with congestive heart failure. Which *three* of the following would you have ready by the bed

A. a bed elevator
B. a bed table
C. oxygen apparatus
D. suction apparatus
E. a bed cradle
F. a drip stand

In each of questions 7–13 there is only ONE correct answer. You have to choose this, so write A, B, C, etc., ONLY.

7. In congestive heart failure the organs of the body become *congested*. Does this mean

   A. that they do not receive enough blood
   B. that they are too full of blood

8. A patient with congestive heart failure has oedema (swelling) of the feet and ankles. Which other part is likely to be oedematous (swollen) also

   A. the face
   B. the neck
   C. the hands
   D. the sacrum

9. With this patient, the two pressure areas needing *most* attention would be

   A. elbows and heels
   B. heels and sacrum
   C. sacrum and hips
   D. spine and shoulder blades

10. As far as this patient's diet is concerned, would you give her

   A. ordinary diet
   B. high-calorie diet
   C. small helpings of anything she fancied
   D. low-protein diet
   E. nourishing fluids only

11. Is this patient more likely

   A. to have diarrhoea
   B. to be constipated

12. In attending to her sanitary needs, which of the following do you consider the most suitable

   A. a commode
   B. a sani-chair
   C. a bedpan

13. If this patient were rude and disagreeable to you, would you

   A. think that she was naturally a disagreeable type of person
   B. think that she had taken a dislike to you personally
   C. think that her brain was suffering from lack of oxygen
   D. be afraid that you had done something to annoy her

Now correct your answers from the notes on the pages 27–9.

ANSWERS AND NOTES ON REVISION QUIZ

For questions 1–6 count marks as shown.

1. A = pulmonary artery; B = superior vena cava
C = right atrium (*or* auricle); D = inferior vena cava
E = right ventricle; F = aorta
G = pulmonary veins; H = left atrium (*or* auricle)
I = left ventricle

Count 1 mark for each part correctly named.

Total = 9 marks.

2. Superior vena cava (B), inferior vena cava (D) and pulmonary veins (G) are the vessels carrying blood *to* the heart (1 mark for each one correct = 3 marks).

These vessels enter the atria (*or* auricles): all blood *entering* the heart enters the atria, the receiving chambers of the heart.

3. The pulmonary artery (A) and aorta (F) carry blood *from* the heart (1 mark for each one correct = 2 marks).

These start from the ventricles, the pumping chambers which pump blood out.

4. The pulmonary veins (G) and the aorta (F) carry *oxygenated* blood (1 mark for each one correct = 2).

The *left* side of the heart contains only oxygenated blood. This enters the left atrium by the pulmonary veins, passes into the left ventricle, and is pumped out through the aorta, as shown in the diagram below.

5. The superior and inferior venae cavae (B, D) and pulmonary artery (A) carry *deoxygenated* blood (1 mark for each one correct = 3).

The *right* side of the heart contains only deoxygenated blood. This returns from the body by the venae cavae into the right atrium, passes into the right ventricle, and is pumped out through the pulmonary artery, as shown in the diagram below.

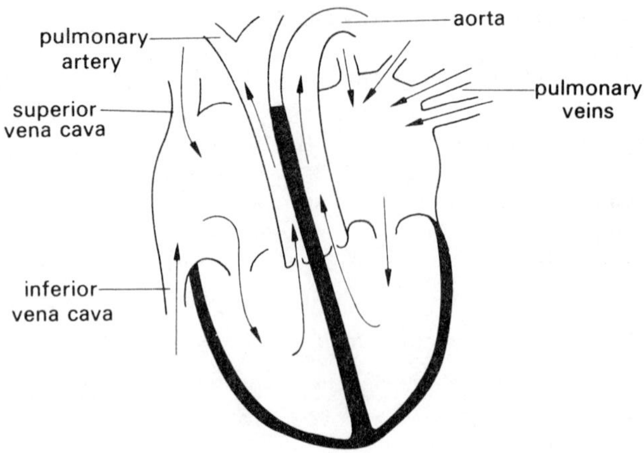

6. B, C and E (1 mark for each one correct = 3 marks).

   A. A *bed-table* (with a pillow on it). The patient is very breathless and may only be able to breathe when sitting upright. Leaning forward on to a bed-table helps: it makes it easier to expand the chest.

   C. *Oxygen apparatus*. Oxygen given occasionally may relieve the patient.

   E. A *bed cradle*. Feet and ankles are usually swollen and feel heavy; this takes the weight of the bedclothes off them.

For questions 7–13 count TWO marks for each correct answer.

Correct answer

7. B. *Congestion* means that the organs are too full of blood. When the heart fails to pump efficiently, it cannot empty, and therefore cannot take all the blood trying to get back into it. It is like congestion of traffic: the hold-up in the heart holds up the blood in all the organs. Congestion in the *lungs* causes breathlessness; in the lower parts of the body (feet and legs) it causes oedema (swelling), as fluid seeps out through the overloaded capillaries.

8. D. Oedema is a collection of fluid in the tissues. This fluid collects in the parts of the body which are lowest. If a patient is on his feet, this will be in the feet and ankles, and then in the legs. If he is lying in bed, fluid will collect in the sacral region, which is then the lowest part.

9. B. Heels and sacrum, where there is oedema, are most liable to develop bedsores.

10. C. Because of congestion in the stomach and abdomen, patients with heart failure usually have a poor appetite and get indigestion. Their appetites need tempting with small amounts of something which they like. They should not have too much fluid.

11. B. All the organs are congested, and this interferes with their normal working. The patient is likely to be constipated.

12. A. A commode is most suitable. Sitting on a bedpan causes much more strain; although the patient will need help from two nurses to be put on a commode, she will be more comfortable in a sitting position.

13. C. Patients with congestive heart failure are often very irritable, and sometimes confused, especially at night, because their brains are getting too little oxygen. The blood congesting the brain is *deoxygenated* blood.

    As their condition improves, they will often be seen to be perfectly reasonable and pleasant people normally.

Maximum Total=36 marks.

Your score will show you how well you have done. Do any more revision which you think you need BEFORE attempting the question on the page opposite.

QUESTION

Without looking back or consulting any book, write the answer to the question on this page. You should not take more than 40 minutes to plan and write your answer.

Mrs Jenkins, aged 45, is admitted to your ward with congestive heart failure.

(a) Draw a large, labelled diagram showing the circulation of blood through the heart.

(b) What symptoms is Mrs Jenkins likely to have, and what nursing measures could you take to relieve them?

When you have finished your answer, and not before, turn over and correct it by the 'model answer' overleaf.

MODEL ANSWER

(a) *Diagram* (15 marks)

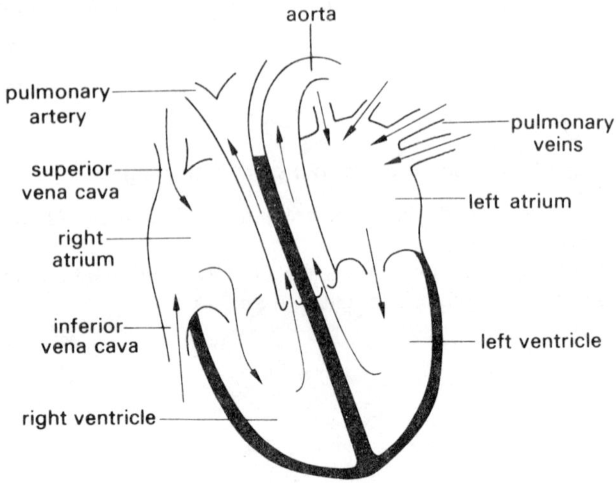

Count marks as follows: 1 mark each for right atrium, left atrium, right ventricle and left ventricle shown correctly = 4; 1 mark for superior vena cava entering right atrium; 1 mark for inferior vena cava entering right atrium; 1 mark for pulmonary veins entering left atrium; 1 mark for pulmonary artery leaving right ventricle; and 1 mark for aorta leaving left ventricle (to get a mark you *must* have shown the blood vessel entering or leaving the correct part of the heart). Then count 6 marks for showing correctly by means of arrows the circulation of blood through the heart.

(b) *Symptoms of congestive heart failure* (85 marks)

Mrs Jenkins will be very breathless (*or* have dyspnoea) (2), and may only be able to breathe sitting upright (2). She will need to be well supported by pillows (2), and should be given a bed-table with a pillow on it (2) so that she can lean forward, as this makes breathing easier (1). The ward should be well ventilated, as she will feel in need of fresh air (2); but she must not be in a draught (1), and should wear a bedjacket to keep her warm (2). Oxygen apparatus should be ready by the bed, as occasional oxygen may give her relief (2). She may be more comfortable if she can have a special cardiac bed, of which the foot can be lowered, so that she is in a sitting position (2).

She must be spared all unnecessary effort, as this will increase her breathlessness (4). Her locker should be where she can reach it easily (2), and she must be washed and helped with her toilet (2) and with her meals (2). As her condition improves she will be allowed to do more, so long as this does not make her breathless (2). Visitors should be asked not to tire or worry her (2).

Her feet and legs may be very oedematous (2) and feel heavy; and the bedclothes should be kept from pressing on them by means of a bed cradle (2). Her sacrum also may be oedematous (2), and she should be given an air-ring, ripple mattress or sheepskin so that it does not become sore (2 for any one). Her sacrum and heels especially will need regular attention to prevent pressure sores (2); they should be kept clean (1) and dry (1), and powdered regularly (1). Her position should be changed as far as possible every two hours (2).

Her appetite will probably be poor (2), and she may have indigestion (2). She should be given small helpings (2) of any food which she fancies (2), without too much to drink with it (2).

She may also be constipated (2). The nurse should watch for this (1) and be ready to give her suppositories (2), or aperients if they are ordered (2). It will be easier for her to use a commode than a bedpan (2), and she will need helping out of bed for this by two nurses (2).

She may sleep badly (2). The nurse should make sure she is as comfortable as possible before settling her for the night (2), and that her sheets are not damp or wrinkled (2). She may get irritable (2), and may become confused at night (2). She will need to be treated with patience and consideration (2); and a shaded light should be left on over her bed at night if she is confused (2).

As various drugs will play an essential part in relieving her symptoms, the nurse must make sure that they are given punctually (3).

Medical Nursing

5 HEART ATTACK

REVISION QUIZ

In each of the following questions there is only ONE correct answer. You have to choose this; so write A, B, or C, etc., ONLY.

1. When a patient is admitted as an emergency with a 'heart attack', do you understand

   A. that he has a cerebral thrombosis
   B. that he has a coronary thrombosis
   C. that he has congestive heart failure
   D. that he has had a fainting attack

2. Typically, is the patient who comes in with a heart attack

   A. an elderly man
   B. an elderly woman
   C. a middle-aged man
   D. a middle-aged woman

3. Is the main symptom of this condition

   A. sudden and persistent pain in the chest
   B. pain in the chest on exertion
   C. sudden unconsciousness
   D. breathlessness
   E. swelling of the ankles

4. On admission, is the patient with a severe heart attack likely to have

   A. a high blood pressure and slow pulse
   B. a high blood pressure and rapid pulse
   C. a low blood pressure and slow pulse
   D. a low blood pressure and rapid pulse

5. Is the reason for attaching a patient to a *cardiac monitor*

   A. to show changes in the rhythm of the heart beat
   B. to show changes in the degree of shock
   C. to stimulate the heart by electricity
   D. to raise his blood pressure

6. A patient who has had a heart attack may be given an intravenous infusion. Is its purpose

   A. to give blood because he is anaemic
   B. to raise his blood pressure
   C. to increase his fluid intake

7. A patient who was admitted a few days ago with a heart attack has an executive job. He is feeling much better, but is worried about a contract which he was in the middle of negotiating. Would it be best

   A. for him to be told to forget about it
   B. for him to be allowed to do some work while in hospital
   C. for his employer to be asked to come and see him

8. After being discharged from hospital, will this patient be able to go back to work

   A. immediately
   B. after about two weeks' convalescence
   C. after about three months' convalescence

9. He lives a mile from his place of employment. Will he be advised

   A. to walk to work
   B. to drive to work
   C. to go by 'bus

Now correct your answers from the notes on pages 37 and 38.

ANSWERS AND NOTES ON REVISION QUIZ

Count TWO marks for each correct answer.

Correct answer

1. B. *'Heart attack' usually means a coronary thrombosis (or* myocardial infarction).

   As shown in the diagram, a branch of the coronary arteries becomes obstructed by a clot of blood or otherwise blocked. This cuts off the blood supply to part of the muscle wall of the heart.

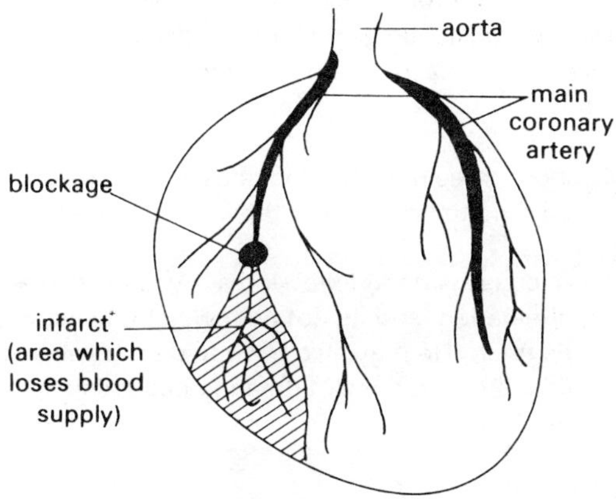

2. C. Most frequently a middle-aged man, very often in a responsible position, with business worries, etc.

3. A. Very severe pain in chest, spreading to neck and down the left arm. The patient may previously have had similar pain on exertion which passes off; but this time it does not pass off.

4. D. Low blood pressure and rapid pulse. Myocardial infarction can cause severe shock.

5. A. The monitor shows changes in the rhythm of the heart. The normal pattern traced by the light on the oscilloscope screen changes if the rhythm of the heart changes. One of the main dangers in the period immediately after a myocardial infarction is that the heart will suddenly stop (cardiac arrest), or that a change in rhythm will

prevent it from pumping out blood; so any change observed on the screen must be reported immediately.

The monitor is a way of taking a continuous electrocardiogram. It picks up electrical currents set up by contractions in the heart muscle. No electricity is passing *from* the machine *to* the patient; it is passing through the machine *from* the patient.

6. B. The intravenous infusion helps to counteract shock by raising the blood pressure. A drug which raises blood pressure such as dopamine may be added to the infusion.

7. C. It is most important for the patient not to worry and to rest. The medical social worker can get in touch with his employer, who is the best person to put his mind at rest by telling him his work is being coped with.

8. C. Probably about three months' convalescence: less or more, of course, according to how severe the infarction was.

9. A. Moderate exercise is good following a myocardial infarction. For one thing, the patient should not gain weight; being overweight is a strain on the heart. He may also have to diet. It will also be good for him to avoid the frustrations of driving or catching 'buses and take things more calmly.

Maximum Total = 18 marks.

Your score will show you how well you have done. Do any more revision which you think you need BEFORE attempting the question on the page opposite.

QUESTION

Without looking back or consulting any book, write the answer to the question on this page. You should not take more than 40 minutes to plan and write your answer.

A sales manager aged 40 years had a sudden heart attack and is admitted to your ward.

(a) What nursing observations will this patient need during the first 24 hours?
(b) How can he be helped to adjust to his illness?

When you have finished your answer, and not before, turn over and correct it by the 'model answer' overleaf.

MODEL ANSWER

(a) *Observations* (60 marks)

The amount of pain and whether it is very severe (5). Whether or not the pain is relieved by the analgesics given (5).

The patient's pulse should be taken and recorded half-hourly (5) and any alterations in its rate or rhythm reported at once (5). If the patient is attached to a monitor, any variations can be seen to occur and the screen should be watched constantly (2).

Blood pressure recordings are made half-hourly (5) so that any fall can be reported at once (3).

His colour should be observed: if he becomes ashen grey, very pale or cyanosed (*or* blue) help should be summoned (4).

Any vomiting should be noted as this may occur due to pain (1).

Urinary output should be charted (2). His urine should be tested as soon as possible and any abnormalities reported and charted (*or* you may say tested for sugar and protein) (3).

The nurse should observe the patient's mental condition: whether he is alert, confused, worried or restless (3 for any TWO suggestions).

It should also be noticed whether the patient eats or drinks: his fluid intake being recorded on his chart (3).

During the night, he may be awake due to his strange surroundings, or because of the pain (2). The amount of sleep he has is also important (3).

If he has an intravenous infusion, nurse should see that it is running satisfactorily and according to instructions with the addition of any drugs which should be checked by a trained nurse (4). The amount given is recorded on the fluid balance chart (2). The infusion site should be checked and his arm comfortably placed on a splint (2).

Any drugs should be recorded (1).

(b) *Adjustment to his illness* (40 marks)

He must be given a proper explanation about his heart attack (5) so that he can be reassured that he will get better if he rests (3).

A social worker or his employer may be asked to visit the patient to ease any worries about his job and offer help of convalescence (4). He may be worried about financial matters and arrangements can often be made to help (2).

His wife should also be seen by the doctor and reassured as much as possible about her husband's future health (3). She should be encouraged to be as cheerful as possible when with her husband (2) and asked not to worry him (2) or allow too many visitors (2).

If he is to have a special diet, full explanation should be given to the patient and his wife and a dietician should be asked to give advice if necessary (*or* you may have specified a weight-reducing or low-cholesterol diet) (4).

If anticoagulant drugs are ordered, he should be given a card to always have with him, and he should be warned about possible bleeding and what to do if it occurs (2).

He may not be able to climb stairs, so before he goes home suitable arrangements may need to be made to have his bed moved downstairs (3); any nursing aids may be borrowed from the Red Cross or social services department (3).

Diversional therapy may be given to maintain his morale (3) (*or* you may suggest books, television, radio, jigsaw puzzles, chess, cards or other suitable pastime).

After a suitable time, he will probably be able to return to work for short periods (1) at first, then longer if his condition allows (1).

Medical Nursing

6 PREPARATION FOR VARIOUS PROCEDURES

REVISION CHART

For this chapter, get together with a friend and fill in the chart below (only write *very brief notes* or you will not have room).

Procedure	*What to tell the patient*	*Position*	*Care during procedure*	*Observations*
Lumbar puncture				
Chest aspiration				
Blood transfusion				
Rectal examination				

Now correct your answers from the notes on pages 44 and 45.

ANSWERS AND NOTES ON REVISION CHART

For convenience these have been written in note form, under headings corresponding with the sections on the chart.

Count marks as indicated.

(a) *Lumbar puncture* (39 marks)

Explanation: That the doctor wishes to take some fluid from his back (2). That he will have a local anaesthetic (like at the dentist) first (2). He will feel no pain, just pressure on his back (2). He must lie very still (2). The nurse will stay with him (2).

Position: On left or right side (2), with knees drawn up (2) and head and shoulders bent forwards (2) so spine is flexed (1). Back should be at edge of bed (2). One pillow for head (2).

Care during procedure: Offer bedpan or urinal before doctor comes (2). Keep covered as much as possible (2). Maintain privacy (2). Reassure (2). May need to keep patient in position by supporting round shoulders (2) (*not* round neck) and knees (1).

Observations: Keep patient lying flat for 12–24 hours (3). Report if he complains of headache (2). Make sure specimens are labelled and taken to laboratory (2).

(b) *Chest aspiration* (45 marks)

Explanation: That the doctor will take some fluid from chest to aid breathing (2). It will not hurt (2) as he will give local anaesthetic (*or* like at the dentist) first (2); he will feel pressure only (1). Must keep very still (1). Nurse will stay with him (2). Should not cough (3). Will give his medicine now to stop him coughing (2) and another dose will be ready if he needs it (2).

Position: Sitting up (2), leaning forward over a bed-table and pillows (2). Should lean slightly away from side to be aspirated to increase space between ribs (3).

Care during procedure: Offer bedpan or urinal before doctor comes (2). Keep covered as much as possible (2). Maintain privacy (2). Reassure (2). If patient needs to cough, give him linctus to sip (2).

Observations: Note and report any change in colour (2). If large amount of fluid aspirated, watch for signs of exhaustion (2) or shock (2). Measure and chart fluid aspirated (2) and send any specimens to laboratory in labelled containers (2). Record half-hourly pulse and respiration chart for as long as instructed (1).

(c) *Blood transfusion* (40 marks)

Explanation: That the doctor is giving him blood to make him feel better (*or* less anaemic) (2). That all he will feel is the prick of the needle (2).

Position: Remove arm from pyjama jacket (*or* nightgown) (3). Place protected pillow under arm (2). Put sphygmomanometer (*or* tourniquet) ready (1). Locker may need moving so patient can reach (1).

Care during procedure: Reassure (2). Check blood with doctor (3). Give bell so he can call for attention (1). When transfusion running, splint arm lightly (2). Make sure what rate of flow is required (2) and what fluid is to follow the blood (2) (*or* whether it is to be taken down).

Observations: That rate of flow is maintained (2). Take temperature, pulse and respirations hourly (2). Observe for skin rashes (2), pain in loin (2) or rigor (2), and report these at once (2). Record fluid balance chart (2). Observe needle area frequently for signs of bruising (2) or inflammation (1).

(d) *Rectal examination* (31 marks)

Explanation: That the doctor is going to examine him internally (2). That it may be uncomfortable (2) but not painful (1). The nurse will stay with him (2).

Position: Left lateral (3); lying on left side, buttocks to edge of bed with knees drawn well up and head on one pillow (4). Trousers down (1). Protective pad under buttocks (2).

Care during procedure: Offer bedpan and/or urinal before doctor comes (2). Reassure (2). Maintain privacy (2). Clean area afterwards (2).

Observations: Notice if patient is in pain during or afterwards (2). Report any faecal incontinence (2) or bleeding (2).

Your score will show you how well you have done. Do any more revision which you think you need BEFORE attempting the question on the page opposite.

QUESTION

Without looking back or consulting any book, write the answer to the question on this page. You should not take more than 40 minutes to plan and write your answer.

How does the nurse prepare *the patient* for *three* of the following procedures:

(a) Lumbar puncture.
(b) Chest aspiration.
(c) Blood transfusion.
(d) Rectal examination.

What observations should the nurse make during and after each of the three procedures?

(*Note to the student*. You have only to answer THREE of the above. It would therefore be sensible to allow 12 minutes for each.)

When you have finished your answer, and not before, turn over and correct it by the 'model answer' overleaf.

MODEL ANSWER

All FOUR parts are answered, although *you* only should have written on THREE.

(a) *Lumbar puncture* (33 marks)

The nurse should explain that doctor wants to take a little fluid from his back for examination (2); that all he will feel is a needle-prick when he is given the local anaesthetic and then some pressure on his back (2). He must lie very still (2). The nurse shuts the window (1) and draws the bed-curtains (1). She will stay with the patient (1).

The patient is offered a bedpan or urinal (2). The nurse removes all except one pillow (1) and helps the patient onto his left or right side (2) with his knees drawn well up (2). His spine should be well rounded and at the edge of the bed (2). His head lies on the pillow and is bent towards his knees (2). When the doctor is ready, the bedclothes are drawn back, his back exposed and his shoulders covered with a small blanket (3).

The nurse may need to support the patient in the correct position by holding him around the shoulders and knees (2). She must make sure the specimen bottles (*or* two specimen bottles) are labelled and sent to the laboratory immediately after (3).

The patient should be kept flat, and quiet, for 12–24 hours afterwards (2), during which time everything is done for him (1). Any headache is reported at once (2).

(b) *Chest aspiration* (34 marks)

The nurse explains that the doctor is going to help his breathing by taking some of the fluid from his chest (2). That this will not hurt and all he will feel is the needle-prick of the local anaesthetic (2) and pressure on his chest (1).

The nurse will stay with him to reassure him (1).

The patient is offered a bedpan or urinal before doctor comes (2). Nearby windows are shut (1) and the bed-curtains drawn (1).

If the patient has a cough, a dose of linctus should be given early enough to suppress it (2) and another dose should be ready in case he needs it while the aspiration is being performed (1).

The patient is helped to sit forward, leaning over a bed-table with pillows on it to support his arms (3). He should lie slightly tilted to the side opposite the one to be aspirated, to increase the space between the ribs (2). His pyjama jacket is removed (1) and his shoulders covered with a small blanket (1).

During and after the procedure, any colour change should be reported (3) or any change in the rate or type of respirations (3). A pulse and respiration chart may be recorded every half-hour (1).

If there is much fluid to be drawn off, the patient may become shocked or very exhausted, and nurse should notice and report this (3).

The aspirated fluid is measured and charted as 'output' (3) and any specimens are sent to the laboratory in labelled containers (1).

(c) *Blood transfusion* (34 marks)

The nurse tells the patient he is going to be given blood to make him feel better (2). He is offered a bedpan or urinal (2).

Nearby windows are closed and curtains drawn round his bed (2).

His arm is removed from his pyjama jacket (2) and rested on a protected pillow (2).

A sphygmomanometer cuff can be put on (*or* a tourniquet) but not tightened (*or* inflated) until the doctor is ready (1). An infusion stand should be put by the bed (1). If necessary the patient's locker can be moved so he can reach his things (1). A blanket should be used to cover his shoulders (1).

The nurse stays with the patient while the doctor commences the transfusion to help reassure him (1). She checks the bottle of blood with doctor to make sure the patient obtains the correct group (*or* compatible blood) (3).

During the transfusion, the patient's temperature, pulse and respirations are taken and recorded hourly (3).

The blood should be seen to be dripping at the correct rate (2) and the needle area inspected frequently for leakage or inflammation (2).

If the patient develops a rash (2), a rigor (2) or pain in his loin (2) the nurse must tell the ward sister at once (1).

When the bottle of blood has been given, the amount is entered on the fluid chart (1) and further instructions sought before the needle is removed (1).

(d) *Rectal examination* (33 marks)

The nurse explains that the doctor is to examine the patient internally and that this will be uncomfortable but not painful (3). She offers him a bedpan and urinal (2). She shuts the window (1) and draws the bed-curtains (1).

The nurse helps the patient into the left lateral position (2), lying on his left side (2), with buttocks to the edge of the bed (2) and his knees drawn well up towards his chin (2). He can have one or two pillows under his head (2). A waterproof sheet and towel (*or* protective pad) is placed under his buttocks (2) and his pyjama trousers pulled down (2).

The nurse stays to reassure and comfort the patient (1).

During the procedure, the nurse watches the patient's face for signs of pain (2) and informs the doctor (2). Afterwards, she should report any pain (1), faecal incontinence (2) or discharge of blood (2) or mucus (2).

Medical Nursing

7 CHRONIC BRONCHITIS: THE RESPIRATORY TRACT

REVISION QUIZ

In each of questions 1–6 there is only ONE correct answer. You have to choose this; so write A, B or C, etc., ONLY.

1. Is the most important cause of chronic bronchitis

   A. atmospheric pollution
   B. excessive smoking
   C. tuberculosis
   D. bacterial infection of the bronchi

2. Are the parts chiefly affected by chronic bronchitis

   A. the trachea and main bronchi
   B. the smaller bronchi and bronchioles
   C. the air spaces in the lungs

3. *Emphysema* often accompanies chronic bronchitis. Is emphysema

   A. pus in the pleural cavity
   B. fluid in the pleural cavity
   C. fluid in the lung
   D. enlargement of the air spaces

4. Which of the following is most likely to be a complication of chronic bronchitis

   A. lobar pneumonia　　B. bronchopneumonia
   C. pleural effusion　　D. pneumothorax

5. Is the heart complication caused by chronic bronchitis

   A. congestive heart failure　　B. coronary thrombosis
   C. mitral stenosis

6. In which of the following ways will oxygen probably be given to a patient with chronic bronchitis

   A. intermittently through a mask
   B. continuously through a mask
   C. by an oxygen tent

Now WRITE the answers to the following questions.

7. Write down two ways in which a patient may be helped to cough up sputum.

8. List all the observations which should be made on an ill patient with chronic bronchitis.

9. *Copy* the diagram below, and name the parts marked A–G.

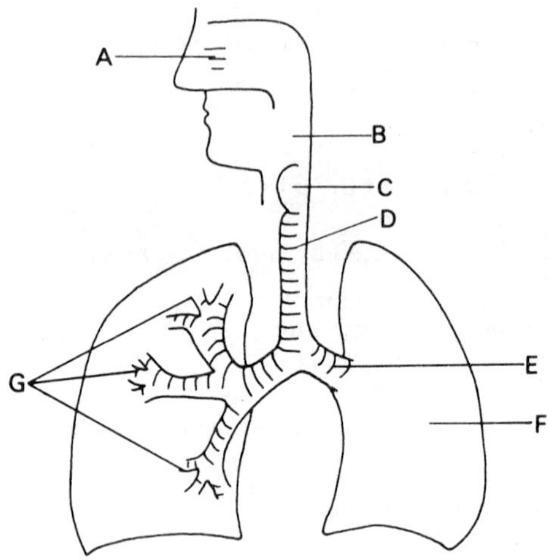

Now correct your answers from the notes on pages 53 and 54.

ANSWERS AND NOTES ON REVISION QUIZ

For questions 1–6 count TWO marks for each correct answer.

Correct answer

1. A. The most important cause is pollution of the atmosphere with smoke and chemicals, especially in a damp climate where fog keeps these suspended in the air.

   Excessive smoking and frequent respiratory infections, such as colds and acute bronchitis are *contributing* causes.

2. B. Chronic bronchitis primarily affects the smaller bronchi inside the lungs and their smallest branches, the bronchioles.

3. D. Emphysema means enlargement of the air-spaces. Their thin walls break down, so that many spaces join together, and blood vessels are destroyed.

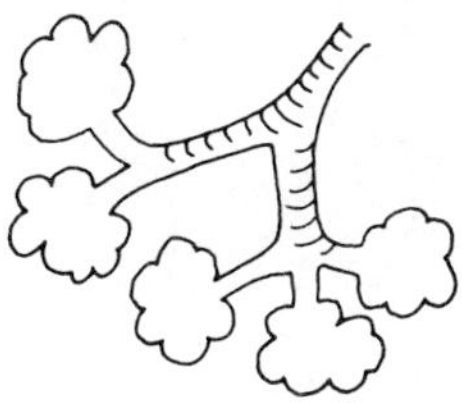

normal

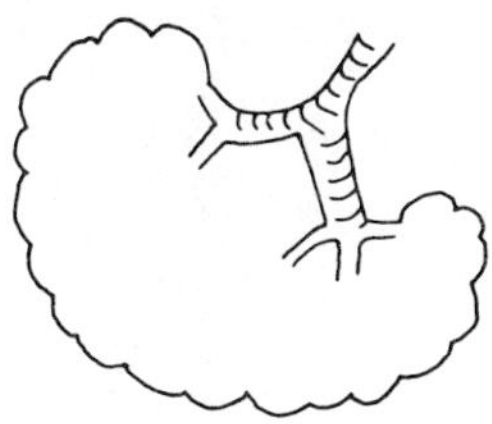

emphysematous

4. B. Bronchopneumonia, *not* lobar pneumonia.

5. A. Congestive heart failure.

   It is often one or both of the above complications which causes admission to hospital. Those who are admitted are frequently very ill indeed.

6. A. These patients are usually given oxygen *intermittently*. Continuous oxygen, especially in a tent, can cause them to stop breathing altogether.

For questions 7–9 count marks as shown.

7. Inhalations: steam (1) or Alevaire (1). These help to loosen sputum. Postural drainage (2).

8. Whether he coughs (1) and brings up sputum (1); character of sputum (1). Breathing (1); whether difficult (1); rate of respiration (1). Pulse rate (1) and any irregularity (1). Rise of temperature (1). Fluid intake and output (1). Bowel actions (1).

9. A = nasal cavity   B = pharynx   C = larynx
   D = trachea   E = main bronchus   F = lung
   G = bronchial tree (*or* smaller bronchi)

   (1 mark for each one correct)

Maximum Total = 32 marks.

Your score will show you how well you have done. Do any more revision which you think you need BEFORE attempting the question on the page opposite.

QUESTION

Without looking back or consulting any book, write the answer to the question on this page. You should not take more than 40 minutes to plan and write your answer.

An elderly man in your ward has chronic bronchitis.

(a) List the causes of this condition.
(b) How should this patient be nursed?
(c) Draw and label a simple diagram of the respiratory tract.

When you have finished your answer, and not before, turn over and correct it by the 'model answer' overleaf.

MODEL ANSWER

(a) *Causes of chronic bronchitis* (15 marks)

Pollution of the atmosphere (3) by smoke (2) and chemicals (2)
Damp climate (2), causing fog (2)
Excessive smoking (2)
Frequent respiratory infections (*or* frequent colds, coughs, acute bronchitis, etc.) (2)

(b) *Nursing care* (65 marks)

The patient will be suffering from lack of oxygen (1), and will therefore find breathing difficult (1). He should be nursed well propped up in bed (3), with a bedtable (2) with a pillow on it (1) for him to lean on (1). The ward should be well ventilated (2), but warm (2).

He should be persuaded not to smoke (2). He may need to be given low concentration oxygen, 24%–28%, intermittently through a venturi system mask (2).

He must be spared all unnecessary effort (2), so if possible two nurses should attend to him (2) for bedmaking (1), washing (1) and attending to his pressure areas (1). He must not get constipated (2), and may need suppositories (2). It may be easier for him to be helped on to a commode than to use a bedpan (2).

He must be given a sputum carton (2), and must be encouraged to cough to get rid of sputum (2). Steam inhalations or inhalations of trypsin or Alevaire may be given (2 for any ONE of these) to help loosen his sputum (1). Nurses may have to give him postural drainage (2) by elevating the foot of his bed or altering his position frequently (1). It is important to observe whether he coughs (2), how much sputum he is bringing up (2) and whether this is very thick and difficult to bring up (2) or contains blood (1).

He should have light, easily digested food (2), and be helped with his meals (2). Nurses must also see that he drinks enough (2), and a fluid balance chart will probably be kept (2).

The patient's temperature, pulse and respiration will be taken four-hourly (2); the nurse must report rises in temperature (1), or in pulse and respiration rates (1), and any irregularity of the pulse (1). She should notice any change in breathing (1) or in the degree of cyanosis (1).

Any drugs which are ordered must be given punctually (3).

(c) *Respiratory tract* (20 marks)

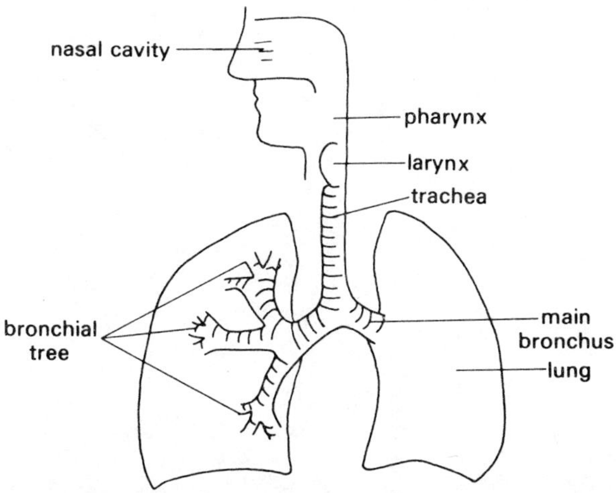

Count TWO marks for each of the parts labelled correctly (= 14 marks). Count SIX marks for the correct size and shape of the organs.

Medical Nursing

8 PNEUMONIA: OXYGEN: THE LUNGS

REVISION QUIZ

In the question at the end of this chapter you are asked about *observations* on a patient. Examiners often ask about 'observations', and there is one common mistake made by students; this is to include *investigations* in their answers. 'Observations' means *what the nurse can observe*, not other investigations which she does *not* make.

In each of questions 1–8 there is only ONE correct answer. You have to choose this; so write A, B, or C, etc., ONLY.

1. Which of the following would be an *investigation* on a patient with pneumonia, *not* an observation

   A. taking his temperature four-hourly
   B. a chest X-ray
   C. looking at his sputum to see if it contained blood
   D. measuring his fluid output

2. If you were told to collect a specimen of sputum to send to the pathological laboratory, would this be

   A. an observation
   B. an investigation

3. Is a patient with pneumonia who is short of oxygen likely to be

   A. cyanosed
   B. flushed
   C. jaundiced
   D. very pale

4. Are this patient's respirations likely to be

   A. slow and difficult
   B. slow and stertorous
   C. shallow and rapid

5. If a patient in an oxygen tent becomes restless and struggles to get out, which of the following should you do first

   A. reassure him and tuck him in firmly
   B. remove the tent for a short time
   C. go to Sister and ask if he can have an injection to sedate him
   D. see if he is too hot or needs a urinal

6. In deciding whether a patient in an oxygen tent is breathing satisfactorily, which of the following is your best guide

   A. you can see regular movements of his chest
   B. his colour is good
   C. he is quiet and appears to be sleeping

7. You can recognize an oxygen cylinder at a glance because

   A. it is black with a white collar
   B. it is black with a green collar
   C. it is black with a red collar

8. Which of the following is true

   A. the pulmonary artery carries deoxygenated blood from the lungs to the heart
   B. the pulmonary artery carries deoxygenated blood from the heart to the lungs
   C. the pulmonary artery carries oxygenated blood from the lungs to the heart
   D. the pulmonary artery carries oxygenated blood from the heart to the lungs

Now WRITE answers to the following questions.

9. List the precautions which must be taken when a patient is being nursed in an oxygen tent.

10. Draw a simple diagram of the lungs and label the main parts.

11. (a) Describe how oxygen is taken in and carbon dioxide excreted inside the lungs.
    (b) Draw a diagram to illustrate this.

Now correct your answers from the notes on pages 61–3.

ANSWERS AND NOTES ON REVISION QUIZ

For questions 1–8 count TWO marks for each correct answer.

Correct answer

1. B. A chest X-ray is an investigation. All the other things were observations. And don't forget, when you answer questions, to put in routine observations such as taking and charting temperature and pulse, or keeping a fluid balance chart.

2. B. Collecting a specimen for the laboratory is not an observation; it is providing the material needed for an investigation in the laboratory.

3. A. Shortage of oxygen is shown by cyanosis, a blue colour due to the bluish colour of deoxygenated blood.

4. C. Respirations in pneumonia are shallow and rapid.

5. D. Patients in oxygen tents are usually very ill, may be mentally confused and feel imprisoned. It is often feeling too hot or needing a bedpan or urinal which makes them restless, but they may not be able to explain.

6. A. Regular movements of the chest tell you that a patient is breathing satisfactorily. The patient in an oxygen tent will usually have a better colour than before; but it is possible for him to stop breathing. So if the patient is very quiet and appears to be sleeping you should look again.

7. A. Black with white collar. It is especially necessary to recognize the different colours on cylinders in theatre, where several kinds are in use.

8. B. You will remember that the pulmonary artery is the only *artery* which carries deoxygenated blood. It takes blood from the right ventricle of the heart to the lungs, as shown below:

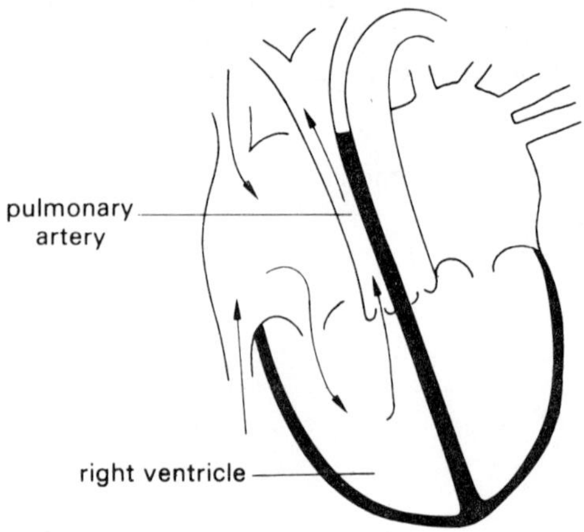

For questions 9–11 count marks as shown.

9. Because of danger of fire (1), matches and lighters must be taken away from all patients (2), and children must not have sparking toys (1). Patients must not wear nylon nightclothes (1), because these cause static electricity (1). Visitors must not smoke (1). A 'No Smoking' notice is put near the tent (1).

To avoid explosions (1) no oil or grease must be put on the apparatus (1).

Care must be taken to use correct cylinders (1). The rate of flow must be kept as ordered (1).

Total= 12 marks.

10. Diagram. Count 1 mark for showing that the lungs are cone-shaped. Count 1 mark for drawing and labelling correctly each of the parts labelled on the diagram.

Total=5 marks.

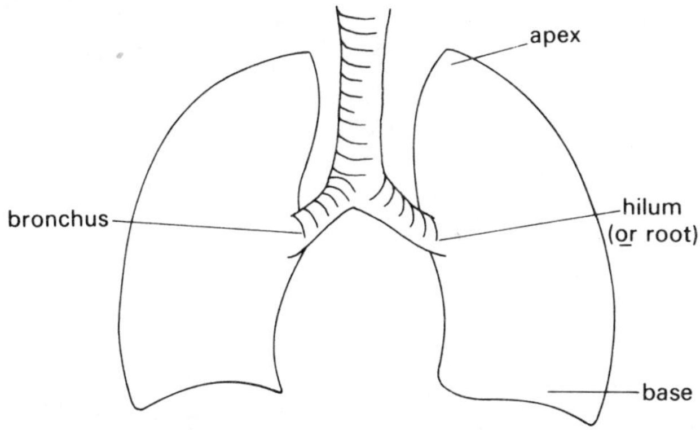

11. (a) Oxygen passes through the thin walls of the air-sacs (*or* alveoli) (1) into the blood in the capillaries (1), which come from the pulmonary artery (1). Carbon dioxide passes out of the blood into the air sacs (1) and is breathed out in expired air (1).

Total=5 marks.

(b) Diagram. Count 5 marks if you have shown the parts labelled, with capillaries surrounding the air-sacs.

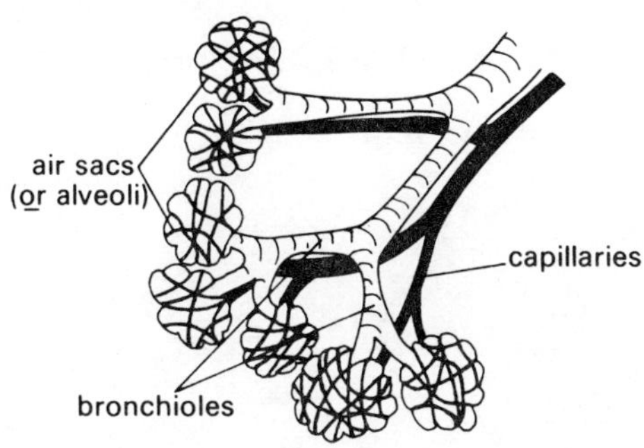

Maximum Total=43 marks.

Your score will show you how well you have done. Do any more revision which you think you need BEFORE attempting the question on the page opposite.

QUESTION

Without looking back or consulting any book, write the answer to the question on this page. You should not take more than 40 minutes to plan and write your answer.

A patient who has pneumonia is having oxygen therapy.

(a) What observations of this patient should be made?
(b) What precautions are necessary when oxygen is in use?
(c) Give a brief description of the lungs.

When you have finished your answer, and not before, turn over and correct it by the 'model answer' overleaf.

MODEL ANSWER

(a) *Observations* (50 marks)

The most important thing is to notice how well the patient is breathing (5), especially by regularly observing the movements of his chest (5). This should be done constantly, as it is possible for a patient to stop breathing while in an oxygen tent (3).

His colour should be noted (2) and whether he is less cyanosed (2).

The nurse should note if the patient is becoming distressed (3). He may be mentally confused (2). She should notice whether he seems to be getting uncomfortably hot (2), or if he is in need of a urinal or bedpan (2).

She should observe whether he coughs (3), and whether he is bringing up sputum (2), and if this is thick and very difficult to bring up (2). The patient should have a sputum carton (1), and the nurse should also notice whether the sputum is streaked with blood (2).

The temperature should be taken four-hourly (2) and charted (1); also the pulse (2) and respiration rates (2). Irregularity of the pulse should be reported (2).

The nurse must notice whether the patient passes urine (2), and report on his output (*or* you may say keep a fluid balance chart) (2). She should also report bowel actions (1).

She must also watch the flowmeter to make sure that the oxygen is flowing at the required rate (2), and that the mask covers the nose and mouth (1).

(b) *Precautions* (20 marks)

To prevent danger of fire (2), matches and lighters should be taken away from all patients (2). Children should not have sparking toys (1). Visitors must not smoke (2), and a 'No Smoking' notice should be displayed (2).

To avoid explosions (1) no oil or grease must be put on cylinders or apparatus (2).

If cylinders are used, the person changing them must be certain they contain oxygen and not some other gas (4). Oxygen cylinders are black with a white 'collar' (1). The oxygen must not flow faster or more slowly than ordered (3).

(c) *The lungs* (30 marks)

(N.B. You can save quite a lot of time by drawing a diagram, as shown below.)

If you have drawn a diagram, count TWO marks for showing the correct shape of the lungs and TWO marks for showing and labelling correctly each of the parts shown.

Total = 10 marks.

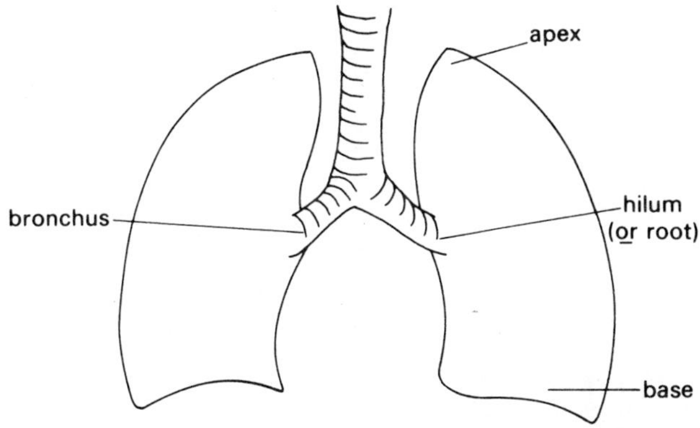

(If you have NOT drawn a diagram, count TEN marks if you have included the following in your description: the lungs are two cone-shaped organs (2), each with an apex at the root of the neck (2), and a base resting on the diaphragm (2). The hilum (*or* root) of the lung is the place where the two main bronchi enter it (4).)

The lungs are covered by a double membrane called the pleura (1). They have a framework of elastic tissue which allows them to expand (2).

Inside the lungs the bronchi divide into smaller branches (1). The smallest branches are the bronchioles (2), which end in air-sacs (*or* alveoli) (2) with very thin walls (1).

The pulmonary artery brings blood to each lung (2). This divides (1), giving off capillaries (2) which surround the air-sacs (2). Oxygen passes from the air in the air-sacs into the blood (2), and carbon dioxide passes from the blood in the capillaries into the air-sacs (2).

Medical Nursing

9 FLUID BALANCE CHARTS AND THE URINARY SYSTEM

REVISION QUIZ

In each of questions 1–6 there is only ONE correct answer. You have to choose this; so write A, B, or C, etc., ONLY.

1. Fluid intake and output are measured in *millilitres* (ml). They can also be expressed in *litres*. If you have a total of 4586 ml, this can also be written as

   A. 45·86 litres
   B. 4·586 litres
   C. 458·6 litres
   D. 0·4586 litres

2. In 2·5 litres there are

   A. 2500 ml
   B. 25 000 ml
   C. 250 ml
   D. 25 ml

3. We lose fluid from the body in urine, through the skin in sweat, and in the moisture in expired air. In normal health, over 24 hours, do we lose, approximately

   A. 1·5 litres in urine, 0·5 litre in sweat and 0·5 litre in expired air
   B. 1 litre in urine, 1 litre in sweat and 1 litre in expired air
   C. 1 litre in urine, 0.5 litre in sweat and 0·5 litre in expired air
   D. 2·5 litres in urine, 0·5 litre in sweat and 0·5 litre in expired air

4. In normal health, does the amount of water in the tissues of the body

   A. vary from day to day according to the amount of fluid taken in
   B. vary according to the amount lost in sweat
   C. remain approximately the same from day to day

5. Reading a *fluid balance chart*, would you expect to see that

   A. the output recorded was more than the recorded intake
   B. the intake recorded was more than the recorded output
   C. the intake and output recorded were the same

6. If a patient is having intravenous fluids only, which of the following *shows best* that he has been given enough fluid over the past 24 hours

   A. the chart shows he has had exactly the amount ordered
   B. the chart shows that he has passed 1·5 litres of urine
   C. the chart shows that he has taken in 2·5 litres of fluid

Now WRITE answers to the following questions.

7. Write down as many conditions as you can for which you have seen fluid balance charts kept.

8. Write down what you would enter on a chart (a) as 'intake' and (b) as 'output'.

9. Draw and label a simple diagram showing the organs of the urinary system.

10. Write down the three main constituents of urine.

Now correct your answers from the notes on pages 71 and 72.

ANSWERS AND NOTES ON REVISION QUIZ

For questions 1–6 count TWO marks for each correct answer.

Correct answer

1. B. 1000 ml = 1 litre; so 4586 ml contain 4 whole litres. The other figures come after the decimal point. 4586 ml, therefore = 4·586 litres.

2. A. 2 litres = 2000 ml; 0·5 litre = 500 ml. So 2·5 litres = 2500 ml.

3. A. Normally the approximate fluid loss is 1·5 litres in urine, 0·5 litre in insensible perspiration and 0·5 litre in expired air during 24 hours.

4. C. The amount of fluid in the tissues remains approximately the same from day to day, because normally what is lost is replaced by what we drink, any excess being excreted in urine. Excessive perspiration simply causes the kidneys to make less urine.

5. B. On a fluid balance chart one is able, with care, to record all the fluid which goes *into* a patient, by mouth or intravenously; but we cannot measure all the *output*, because we cannot measure sweat or the water in expired air. Therefore *on the chart* more intake will normally appear than the amount of output.

6. B. If the patient is passing a satisfactory amount of urine it shows that he is getting enough fluid. If he were *not* getting enough, the kidneys would make less urine. One of their functions is to keep up the balance of water in the tissues. So B. is the best guide to whether the patient is getting enough.

   The patient on intravenous fluids may be very dehydrated, and need much more fluid than a normal person; so his *intake* is not such a good guide.

For questions 7–10 count marks as shown.

7. Conditions you could have mentioned are:

   Kidney disease (*or* any examples of this, such as acute nephritis, chronic nephritis, renal failure, uraemia) (2)

   Dehydration (2)

Conditions which cause dehydration such as excessive vomiting (2) or diarrhoea (2)

Burns (2)

Unconsciousness (2)

8. *Intake:* fluid taken by mouth or nasogastric tube (2), fluid medicines (2) intravenous fluids (2).

   Output: urine (2), vomit (2), gastric aspirations (2), drainage from tubes (2).

9. Your diagram should look like the one shown below. Count 2 marks for drawing and labelling correctly each of the parts shown (=10 marks). Count 2 marks for having the organs approximately the right size and shape.

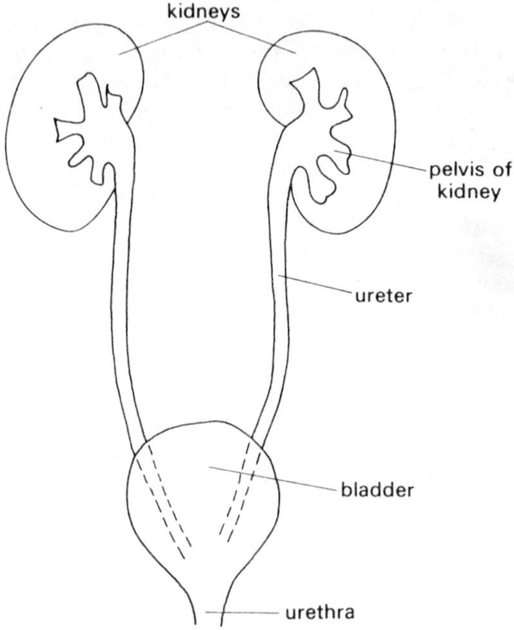

10. Water (2), mineral salts (2) and urea (*or* waste products of protein) (2).

Maximum Total=56 marks.

Your score will show you how well you have done. Do any more revision which you think you need BEFORE attempting the question on the opposite page.

QUESTION

Without looking back or consulting any book, write the answer to the question on this page. You should not take more than 40 minutes to plan and write your answer.

Part of your work in the wards will be involved with fluid balance charts.

(a) What is their purpose?
(b) What is your responsibility with regard to the maintenance of these charts?
(c) Give a brief description of the urinary system.

(*Hint to the student.* In part (c), it will save you a lot of time if you draw a diagram as in the 'Revision questions'; then your description can be much shorter.)

When you have finished your answer, and not before, turn over and correct it by the 'model answer' overleaf.

MODEL ANSWER

(a) *Purpose of fluid balance charts* (35 marks)

Fluid balance charts are kept in order to compare accurately the amount of fluid which a patient takes in with the amount he loses (3). They show whether he is getting sufficient fluid (1) and whether he is passing enough urine to get rid of his waste products (2).

As the loss of fluid in sweat and expired air cannot be measured, the measured output on the chart will normally be less than the measured intake (1).

Charts may be kept:

1. For patients with kidney disease (3). The chart shows whether a patient is passing too little urine (1) and whether or not his output is improving (2).
2. For patients who are dehydrated (3), for example through vomiting (1), diarrhoea (1), or especially burns (2). These patients will probably be having intravenous fluids (2); and must have enough fluid to keep the urinary output for 24 hours up to about 1·5 litres (2). If less is passed, the chart shows the doctor that the patient needs more fluid; if the output is satisfactory, he is getting enough (2).
3. For unconscious patients (3) or those who are very ill (1) or old (1), to make sure they are being given enough fluid (2) and also are passing enough urine to excrete waste products (2).

(b) *The nurse's responsibilities* (30 marks)

The nurse's responsibilities are

1. To make sure that charts are filled in correctly (1) with patients' names (1), dates (1) and times (1).
2. To measure all fluid intake and output accurately (2), and record measurements immediately (2).
3. To enter on the intake side (1) fluid taken by mouth (1), including medicines (1). Amounts of intravenous fluid (2) must be entered as soon as each container is finished (2).
4. To enter on the output side (1) all urine passed (2), gastric aspirations (2), vomit (2) and any drainage from tubes (2).
5. Total intake and output must be added up every 12 hours at the same times each day (2).
6. If urinary output is getting less (2), or if a patient is not passing urine (2) this must be reported to the sister or the doctor.

(c) *The urinary system* (35 marks)

Count ONE mark for drawing and labelling correctly each of the parts shown (=5 marks). Count TWO marks for having the organs approximately the right size and shape.

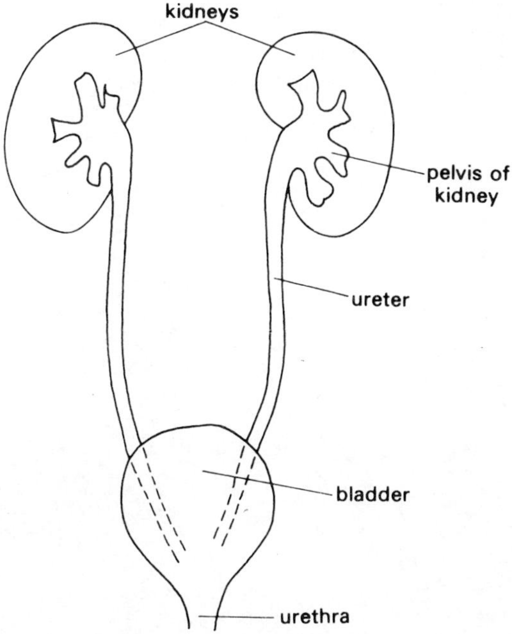

The *kidneys* make urine (2), which contains water (2), mineral salts (2) and urea (*or* waste products of protein) (2). These are removed from the blood circulating round the kidneys (2). Urine is collected in small tubes (1) which lead into the pelvis of the kidney (1). It then flows down the *ureters* (2) into the *bladder* (2). It remains in the bladder until it is passed (2) through the *urethra* (2). This happens when sphincter muscles at the neck of the bladder relax (1).

Functions of the urinary system are

1. To remove unwanted substances from the blood (2) and so to keep its composition correct (1).
2. To remove excess water (2) and maintain the correct amount in the body tissues by excreting more, or less, urine (*or* to regulate the water balance of the body) (2).

Medical Nursing

10 DIABETES MELLITUS

REVISION QUIZ

In each of questions 1–10 there is only ONE correct answer. You have to choose this; so write A, B, or C, etc., ONLY.

1. A diabetic patient cannot use the carbohydrate foods which he eats because of lack of insulin. Which *one* of the following foods contains no carbohydrate at all

   A. bread B. carrots C. bananas
   D. milk E. butter F. chocolate
   G. apple pie

2, Which *one* of the following would be restricted in the diet of a diabetic

   A. pickles B. white sauce C. tomatoes
   D. coffee E. cabbage F. salt
   G. beef steak

3. In a *normal* diet, the daily amount of carbohydrate would be about

   A. 2000 g B. 400 g C. 150 g
   D. 100 g E. 50 g

4. In a diabetic's diet, the daily amount of carbohydrate might be restricted to about

   A. 1000 g B. 500 g C. 150 g
   D. 50 g E. 10 g

5. The amount of carbohydrate in a teaspoonful (5 ml) of sugar or glucose is about

   A. 5 g B. 20 g
   C. 50 g D. 100 g

6. The body normally produces insulin in the pancreas. Is it described as

   A. an enzyme B. an internal secretion
   C. a digestive juice

7. Does insulin

   A. prevent there being any sugar in the blood
   B. reduce the amount of sugar in the blood
   C. increase the amount of sugar in the blood

8. A diabetic is 'stabilized' when a correct diet has been found for him, and the correct dose of insulin to balance it. We know when he is stabilized by testing his urine. When he is stabilized, should this contain

   A. no sugar or acetone
   B. a trace of sugar and a trace of acetone
   C. no acetone and a trace of sugar

9. There are various kinds of insulin. *Soluble* insulin is generally used while a patient is being stabilized. Is this because

   A. it contains more units than other kinds of insulin
   B. it contains fewer units
   C. it acts for a longer period than other kinds
   D. it acts more quickly than other kinds

10. If you noticed a patient who was being stabilized sweating and acting strangely, should you

   A. give him some sugar or glucose immediately
   B. give him some insulin immediately
   C. send for the doctor
   D. reassure him and do nothing else

Now WRITE answers to the following questions.

11. Make a list of all the things a new diabetic must know about if he is to live a normal life and keep well when he returns home.

12. List as many possible complications of diabetes as you can.

Now correct your answers from the notes on pages 79 and 80.

ANSWERS AND NOTES ON REVISION QUIZ

For questions 1–10 count TWO marks for each correct answer.

Correct answer

1. E. Butter contains only fat. All the other foods listed contain either starch or some form of sugar.

2. B. White sauce is made with flour, containing starch. None of the other foods contains any carbohydrate to speak of. Only the *milk* in coffee would be rationed.

3. B. 400 g is about the amount which a normal person's diet might contain.

4. C. A diabetic's carbohydrate intake is restricted usually to something between 120 and 200 g daily; so 150 g is the only possible figure in this list.

5. A. 1 teaspoon (5 ml) of sugar or glucose contains about 5 g of carbohydrate

6. B. An internal secretion, poured directly into the blood.

7. B. Insulin allows the sugar in the blood to be used, and therefore *reduces* the amount. We must have some sugar in the blood all the time to produce heat and energy. Insulin keeps the amount down to the correct level.

8. C. There should be no acetone or sugar in urine. Recent advances show that complications are minimised by this status.

9. D. Soluble insulin is the quickest acting kind. It is safer during stabilization, because reaction to an overdose is seen immediately. Other kinds, such as Protamine Zinc insulin, act over a longer period, and are used later so that the patient only needs one injection a day. Whatever kind of insulin he has, the number of *units* per day will be the same once he is stabilized.

10. A. Sweating and acting strangely are signs that the insulin has reduced the blood sugar too much; so he should be given some sugar or glucose immediately.

For questions 11 and 12 count marks as shown.

11. He must understand his diet (1) and which foods are restricted (1); how to measure insulin (1), how to inject himself with it (1) and how to sterilize syringe (1); how to test urine (1). He must know that he should take sugar if he has an insulin reaction (1) and should carry some about with him (1) and also always carry his 'diabetic card' (1); that he must always eat his full ration of carbohydrate (1), and can replace each 5 g with 1 teaspoon (5 ml) sugar if he cannot eat (1); that he must always take his insulin (1) and should go to his doctor if his urine contains much sugar or acetone (1), or if he is ill (1).

    Total= 14 marks.

12. Count ONE mark each for any 6 of the following: diabetic coma; sepsis (*or* example such as boils, carbuncles, etc.), gangrene; arteriosclerosis; cataract; retinitis; peripheral neuritis; chronic renal failure.

    Total=6 marks.

Maximum Total=40 marks.

Your score will show you how well you have done. Do any more revision which you think you need BEFORE attempting the question on the page opposite.

QUESTION

Without looking back or consulting any book, write the answer to the question on this page. You should not take more than 40 minutes to plan and write your answer.

A young person in your ward has been diagnosed as suffering from diabetes mellitus.

(a) What treatment may be ordered for him in hospital until he is stabilized?
(b) What instructions and advice should be given when he is discharged?
(c) List the possible complications which can occur as a result of diabetes.

(*Hint to the student*. Notice the word 'List' in (c). You need not *explain* the complications; just make a list of them.)

When you have finished your answer, and not before, turn over and correct it by the 'model answer' overleaf.

MODEL ANSWER

(a) *Treatment in hospital* (55 marks)

A diet will be ordered in which the amount of carbohydrate is restricted (3) to 120–200 g (any figure within these limits is all right) (2). Other kinds of food are not restricted (2).

At the same time a trial dose of insulin will be prescribed (3). This will be soluble insulin at first (2), given 20 minutes before each main meal (2).

The patient's urine will be tested for sugar (2) and acetone (*or* ketones, *or* diacetic acid) (2) every four hours (2). If it continues to contain an excess of sugar, the number of units of insulin will be increased (2) until the urine contains only a trace (2). This shows that enough insulin is being given for the patient to use up nearly all the carbohydrate in his diet (2). If the patient gets very hungry, his diet can be increased (1), and the dose of insulin increased to balance it (2).

Once the patient has been stabilized (*or* the right diet and dose of insulin have been found), a long-acting insulin (*or* Protamine Zinc insulin or other example) is given instead of soluble (2), so that he will only need one injection a day (2). This is given in the morning before breakfast (2).

While in hospital, the patient is taught the importance of his diet (1), and is given a diet sheet (1) showing which foods are restricted and how much of them he may have (2), and which foods he may eat without restriction (1).

He is also taught how to test his urine for sugar and acetone (4), and should do this every morning before having his insulin (2).

He learns how to measure his insulin (2), how to give himself injections (2) and sterilize the equipment (1), and how to vary the site of the injection each day (1).

He may be allowed to have a mild insulin reaction, so that he knows what it feels like (1); he is told that if he has one he should take some sugar immediately (2).

(N.B. You may have put some of the things which the patient is taught in the next part of the question. If you have, you can count the marks as above; although really these should be taught *before* the patient is discharged.)

(b) *Instructions on discharge* (35 marks)

The patient should be reminded of the importance of the routine he has learned of testing his urine (1), giving himself his insulin (1) and keeping to his diet (1); and told that if he does this he will be able to live a normal life (3).

He is told that he must never miss his insulin (3), and must always eat his full ration of carbohydrate in order to balance it (3). If he is ill and cannot eat, he can take 1 teaspoonful of sugar for each 5 g of carbohydrate in his diet (3).

He will be given urine testing equipment (2), insulin syringe and needles (2) and a supply of the correct type of insulin (2). He will be given an appointment to attend the diabetic clinic (2); and is also told to consult his own doctor if his urine contains more than 1% of sugar (2), or acetone (1), or if he has any other illness (3). He is given a card which he must carry, saying he is a diabetic on insulin (3); and should be told to carry some sugar with him always in case of an insulin reaction (3).

(c) *Complications* (10 marks)

Diabetic coma; sepsis (*or* examples, such as boils, carbuncles, septic fingers); gangrene; arteriosclerosis; cataract; retinitis; peripheral neuritis; chronic renal failure.

Count TWO marks each for any 5 of the above (=10 marks).

General Nursing

11 THE RESPONSIBILITIES OF A NURSE

REVISION QUIZ

In each of questions 1–6 there is only ONE correct answer. You have to choose this; so write A, B or C, etc., ONLY.

1. When answering the ward telephone, should you first say

   A. 'Hullo, who is that speaking?'
   B. 'This is ward X, Nurse Jones speaking.'
   C. 'Hold the line, I'll call Sister.'
   D. 'What do you want?'

2. On answering the telephone a laboratory technician tells you he has a report that Sister is waiting for. She is accompanying the doctor on a ward round. Would you

   A. Interrupt the doctor's round and give her the message verbally
   B. Write the report down and pass it to the doctor
   C. Leave the message on a pad in Sister's office
   D. Ask the technician to telephone back later
   E. Excuse yourself and pass the written message to Sister.

3. A near relative telephones to ask about an ill patient's condition. Should you

   A. Refer to the Kardex report and give an answer to the relative
   B. Ask Sister to come to the telephone
   C. Ask the caller to telephone later when the doctor will have seen the patient
   D. Tell her that the patient 'is as comfortable as can be expected'.

4. You are admitting an elderly, deaf patient. To find the best way of communicating with him, would you

   A. Shout at him to try and make him hear
   B. Talk to the relative and not to the patient
   C. Write everything down for him to read
   D. Ask the relative if he uses a hearing aid.

5. Which of the following would be of most help to this deaf patient during his convalescence

A. Talking books
B. Speech therapy
C. Visitors
D. Another deaf patient
E. Wireless
F. Television

6. What is meant by the term 'dyspnoea'. Is it difficulty in

A. breathing
B. passing urine
C. speaking
D. swallowing

Now WRITE the answer to the following question.

7. Write down a list of ways in which a nurse can help a patient with dyspnoea.

Now correct your answers from the notes on pages 87 and 88.

ANSWERS AND NOTES ON REVISION QUIZ

For questions 1–6 count TWO marks for each correct answer.

Correct answer

1. B. Whenever you answer a telephone it is always correct to give your number first. It can save time as the caller knows at once if he has the wrong number. Sister certainly need not always be called to the 'phone herself but, of course, any message must be taken correctly.

2. E. Sister will obviously want the message before the doctors leave the ward and they may not go into the office. Messages should always be passed to Sister that she can tell the doctor at the right time. This particular message may be difficult to take down, so nurse must ask the technician to spell words she may not be familiar with in order to avoid mistakes which could affect the patient's treatment.

3. B. If Sister is able, she will probably wish to speak to the relative herself. Otherwise she will give you a message to pass on, but she should always be consulted about an ill patient.

4. D. It is best to do this first, as the patient may have brought his hearing aid with him and only needs help in putting it in position. If not, the relative can be asked to bring it in next time she comes. The patient may be able to hear if you speak loudly and slowly to him, but this may disturb other patients and may cause embarrassment to him. Writing things down may be suitable but he may be too ill to bother, may not have his glasses or may be confused. The relative can certainly be of help, but the patient should not be excluded as a deaf person is often suspicious that others are discussing him or treating him as a child.

5. C. His friends and relatives wiil know how best to 'amuse' this patient. Deaf people can often hear a radio if it is tuned correctly and is not too loud for other patients; they also may be able to enjoy television as many are able to lip-read. (You can count ONE mark if you chose wireless or television.)

6. A. Difficulty in passing urine = dysuria
Difficulty in speaking = dysphasia
Difficulty in swallowing = dysphagia

For question 7 count marks as shown for each correct item.

7. Sit the patient upright (3)
Allow him to lean over a bed-table (3)
Put his bed near a window (1)
Give any drugs ordered that will dilate his air passages (3)
Do everything for the patient to spare him any physical effort (2)
Reassure him that you have asked doctor to come to see him (2)
Steam inhalations may help him expectorate and so ease his breathing (4).

Maximum Total = 30 marks.

Your score will show you how well you have done. Do any more revision which you think you need BEFORE attempting the question on the page opposite.

QUESTION

Without looking back or consulting any book, write the answer to the question on this page. You should not take more than 40 minutes to plan and write your answer.

Write short notes on the nurse's responsibilities for:

(a) answering the ward telephone
(b) the elderly patient who is deaf
(c) the relief of dyspnoea

When you have finished your answer, and not before, turn over and correct it by the 'model answer' overleaf.

MODEL ANSWER

(a) *Answering the ward telephone* (33 marks)

This should be done as quickly as possible (2). The name (*or* number) of the ward should be stated (3) and the name of the person answering (4).

If there is a message, this should be written down and read back to the caller (4) and given to the person in charge at once (3). If it is a request to 'ring back', make sure you have the caller's name correct and that the number is known (4).

If it is an enquiry about a patient's condition, the sister or staff nurse should be asked and the message conveyed correctly to the caller (3).

Reports from laboratory or X-ray department must be taken down word-for-word and read back to the caller to avoid mistakes (4). If there is any doubt, or the message cannot be understood, ask the sister or staff nurse to come to the telephone (4).

If the sister or staff nurse is busy, or with a doctor, excuse yourself before giving the message if it cannot wait until she is free (2).

(b) *The elderly deaf patient* (34 marks)

The nurse must try to communicate with him to prevent loneliness (2) and so she can know how to help him (2).

Some deaf patients can lip-read (2), in which case the nurse must speak slowly and carefully so she can be understood (2). Others use a hearing-aid (2) and the nurse must make sure it is in position and switched on before she speaks to the patient (3).

Some deaf people tend to shout as they cannot hear themselves and this may disturb others, especially at night (2). It may be best to write down questions on a pad for the patient to read, especially if they are of a private nature (2) when it may save embarrassment (1). The patient may need to be handed his glasses so he can read the note (1).

Elderly patients may have more difficulty in hospital as voices are strange and there is often background noise (3). Wireless or television sets may have to be made louder than normal, or special headphones may be needed to avoid spoiling other patients' listening or viewing (4).

Relatives may often converse more easily with the patient and they should be allowed in as often as possible if this is so (4).

If the patient has no hearing-aid, the doctor may ask for one to be provided and write the necessary request form which the nurse sends to the appropriate department (2). The nurse can be helpful in encouraging patients to use it as often they are unwilling to try and find it difficult at first to adjust the hearing-aid (2).

(c) *Relief of dyspnoea* (33 marks)

A patient who has breathing difficulties (5) finds respiration easier if he sits upright (2), well supported with pillows (1). This enables the chest to expand freely (1) and allows the diaphragm to move downwards (1).

He may be helped further if a bed-table is placed over the bed with a pillow on it (2) over which the patient may lean (1). He can then use his shoulders to help his breathing (*or* his accessory muscles of respiration) (3).

The patient must be reassured that he will be given treatment by the doctor to help his breathing (2).

If possible the patient's bed should be near a window to allow him more air (2).

Steam inhalations may help the patient to expectorate and this will also help his breathing (2).

The patient should be kept at rest and spared any undue exertion (2); as he is likely to be very frightened, nurse should stay with him until the attack has passed (2).

Any drugs ordered by doctor to dilate the bronchial tree should be given by the nursing staff (2) and their effects reported (2).

Cyanosis (*or* blueness of the extremities) may accompany the dyspnoea when oxygen may be given through a disposable face-mask (*or* Ventimask) (2) at the rate of 4 litres per minute (1).

General Nursing

12 CONTROLLED DRUGS

REVISION QUIZ

In each of questions 1–3 there is only ONE correct answer. You have to choose this, so write A, B or C, etc., ONLY.

1. Are the rules governing the use of 'controlled drugs' laid down

   A. by Act of Parliament
   B. by the hospital authorities
   C. by the Regional Health Authorities

2. Is the reason for drugs being listed as 'controlled drugs'

   A. that they are highly poisonous
   B. that they are habit-forming
   C. that they have dangerous side-effects

3. If you are in charge of the ward and a doctor asks you in an emergency to give him an ampoule of a controlled drug, should you

   A. give him the key of the cupboard
   B. open the cupboard yourself
   C. refuse to let him have the drug
   D. ring the pharmacist

Now WRITE answers to the following questions.

4. From the following list, pick out the five drugs which are 'controlled drugs'

A. atropine	B. butobarbitone	C. cocaine
D. cortisone	E. diamorphine	F. digoxin
G. insulin	H. methadone	J. methyldopa
K. omnopon	L. pethidine	M. phenobarbitone
N. scopolamine		

5. In a few words, say what *mistakes* are made in the following procedure for checking an injection of a controlled drug.

(i) The ward sister unlocks the cupboard.
(ii) She consults the prescription on the patient's drug sheet and selects the correct drug.
(iii) She then sends for the nurse who is to give it, tells her how much has to be given and watches her draw up the dose into a syringe, making sure the dose is correct.
(iv) The sister and nurse then enter particulars in the Controlled Drug Register: date, patient's name, dose and time of giving. They both sign the register.
(v) The nurse then goes and gives the injection, while the sister counts up the stock of the drug which is left and enters it in the register.
(vi) The sister then adds her signature and the time to the prescription on the patient's drug sheet, to show that the drug has been given.

Now correct your answers from the notes on pages 95 and 96.

ANSWERS AND NOTES ON REVISION QUIZ

For questions 1–3 count TWO marks for each correct answer.

Correct answer

1. A. Rules are laid down by Act of Parliament: the Misuse of Drugs Act 1971 which has replaced the former Dangerous Drugs Act.

2. B. These are all habit-forming drugs which cause addiction.

3. B. The person in charge must keep the key; so you open the cupboard yourself, check it with the doctor and record it in the register.

For questions 4 and 5 count marks as shown.

4. The following are controlled drugs. Count TWO marks for each one you have correct

C. cocaine	E. diamorphine (heroin)	
H. methadone	K. omnopon	L. pethidine

5. *Mistakes:* These drugs must be checked *by two people* from start to finish; so

The nurse should have been with the sister when she got out the drug, and *both* should have read the prescription on the patient's drug sheet (2), and should have checked the drug (2) and the patient's name (2).

They should also have made sure and agreed that the dose had not been given already (2).

They are right next to fill in date, patient's name and the dose in the Controlled Drugs Register; but they should not add the time (2) or their signatures until after the dose has been given (2).

They must also *both* count up the stock of the drug left when it is entered in the register (2).

The sister as well as the nurse is responsible for seeing that the dose is given to the right patient; so both should go to the bedside to check this (2).

The nurse, rather than the sister, should have signed the drug sheet to show that the drug had been given (2). (Especially as the sister in this case had not seen it given!)

Maximum Total= 34 marks.

Your score will show you how well you have done. Do any more revision which you think you need BEFORE attempting the question on the page opposite.

QUESTION

Without looking back or consulting any book, write the answer to the question on this page. You should not take more than 40 minutes to plan and write your answer.

(a) What is a controlled drug? Give two examples.
(b) Describe the rules which are observed in hospital for the checking and administration of controlled drugs.

When you have finished your answer, and not before, turn over and correct it by the 'model answer' overleaf.

MODEL ANSWER

(a) *A controlled drug* (20 marks)

A controlled drug is one which is habit-forming (*or* causes addiction) (5), and which is listed in the Misuse of Drugs Act (5). (N.B. If you have said 'controlled by an Act of Parliament' only, count 3 marks).

Examples are derivatives of opium, such as morphine, omnopon, diamorphine (*or* heroin); cocaine; pethidine; methadone.

Count FIVE marks for *any two* (= 10 marks).

(b) *Rules for checking and administration* (80 marks)

In hospital these drugs must be kept locked up (2) in a special cupboard which contains nothing else (2). The key must be kept on the person of the nurse in charge of the ward (5), and she must open the cupboard herself and give out the drugs when they are needed (3).

Controlled drugs may not be administered unless a doctor has ordered the dose in writing (5) on the patient's drug sheet (2).

Each dose must be checked by two people (5); one is usually the nurse in charge (1) and the other the nurse who is to give it (1). Both check the patient's name on the drug sheet (3) and the prescription (3), and make sure the dose has not been given already (2). The prescription is compared with the label on the container (3); both nurses must agree that they have the correct drug (3) and dose (3). If a dose has to be measured from a stock mixture or solution, both must check that the amount is correctly calculated (3).

The drug sheet is taken to the bedside (2), and both nurses must check that it is given to the right patient (2). Unless the patient is unconscious or confused, he is addressed by name so that he can respond to it (2).

Every dose is recorded in a special Controlled Drugs Register (5), which has a section for each different drug (2). The date (2), patient's name (2) and dose (2) are entered when the drug is checked (1). The amount of the drug left in stock is also recorded (2). Immediately after giving the drug, both nurses sign the register (2), entering the time (2). The nurse who gave it also signs the patient's drug sheet (2), adding the time (1).

The pharmacy keeps a register of all controlled drugs issued to wards and departments (2); and the ward register has to be taken to the pharmacy when stock is ordered (2), so that the amount given can be checked with the amount issued (1).

Paediatric Nursing

13 CARE OF CHILDREN IN HOSPITAL

REVISION QUIZ

In each of questions 1–4 there is only ONE correct answer. You have to choose this; so write A, B or C, etc., ONLY.

1. When giving young Jimmy a dose of medicine he does not like, would you tell him

   A. to drink it at once or you will be very cross
   B. you will give him a sweet when he has taken it
   C. that Mummy will only come to see him if he drinks it
   D. that it tastes very nice

2. If Jimmy still refuses his medicine, would you

   A. sit him on your lap and talk to him first
   B. fill the glass with water to make a longer drink
   C. drink some yourself to show him how nice it is
   D. tell him he can go home when he has taken it

3. It is Jimmy's first night in hospital. When settling him down for the night, would it be *best* to

   A. ask his parents to leave without saying 'goodnight'
   B. let his mother put him to bed as she does at home
   C. bath him, give a drink and turn the light out
   D. let his mother bath him ready for the nurse to tuck him up

4. Sally has just vomited. Should you *first*

   A. go and fetch a vomit bowl
   B. tell her she should have called you before she was sick
   C. report the matter to sister
   D. comfort her and tell her she will soon feel better

Now WRITE answers to the following questions.

5. List the things which may frighten a small child on his first night in hospital.

6. List *in the correct order*, the steps you would take to deal with a child who has just vomited over her bed.

Now correct your answers from the notes on pages 101 and 102.

ANSWERS AND NOTES ON REVISION QUIZ

For questions 1–4 count TWO marks for each correct answer.

Correct answer

1. B. Always try the gentle art of persuasion first, if possible with a reward, such as a sweet. Never use threats or tell lies to children as they cease to trust you. Any hint that parents will only 'love him' if he is good, is psychologically unacceptable and may lead to abnormal behaviour.

2. A. You should never make medicines larger in quantity than is absolutely necessary—it is difficult enough to get a child to take a small dose. Answer C is a dangerous practice, though a nurse may *pretend* to a small child to do this. It may be all right to tell a child he can go home 'tomorrow' if, in fact, he *can*.

3. B. In most children's wards, today, mothers do as much of the nursing of their small children as possible. Some mothers may have difficulties with other small children at home, but most will make suitable arrangements in order to be with the sick child at least until he is asleep.

4. D. All the other things can be left until this has been done; another nurse can fetch a bowl in case she vomits again. Answer 'B' may imply that you are cross with the child—children often vomit without warning, anyway.

For questions 5 and 6 count marks as shown.

5. Being without his mother (1). Strange faces (1). Strange noises (1). The dark (1). Feeling ill or in pain (1). Being thirsty and not understanding whom to call (1). He may be old enough to worry about requiring urinal or bedpan (*or* about soiling the bed) (1). He may know he is to have an operation and is afraid (1). He may suddenly wake in the night, not know where he is, and be afraid to call (1). He may be physically uncomfortable: too hot, cold, hungry and not know what to do about it (1 for any ONE suggestion).

6. Comfort her *first* (see above).

   Explain that it is because she is not well, that you are not cross and the 'mess' does not matter (3). That you will soon clear it up (1). Draw the curtains (1). Fetch clean linen and clothing (2) and a bowl of hot water (1). Bring container for soiled linen (1). If possible, take the child to the bathroom and wash or bath her (*or* do this in bed) (2). Help her clean her teeth and use a pleasant-tasting mouthwash (2). Make the bed with clean linen (1). Report to sister (1) whether or not the child's condition seems better or worse (1); the nature of the vomit (1); the amount vomited (1) and whether or not it was related to food, sweets or medicine (1 for any ONE of these suggestions). Leave a vomit bowl and cloth on her locker in case she wants to be sick again (1).

Maximum Total = 38 marks.

Your score will show you how well you have done. Do any more revision which you think you need BEFORE attempting the question on the page opposite.

QUESTION

Without looking back or consulting any book, write the answer to the question on this page. You should not take more than 40 minutes to plan and write your answer.

Your are working in the children's ward. How would you

(a) persuade a child of three to take his medicine
(b) help a child to settle on his first night in hospital
(c) care for a child who has just vomited

When you have finished your answer, and not before, turn over and correct it by the 'model answer' overleaf.

MODEL ANSWER

(a) *How to persuade a child of three to take his medicine* (33 marks)

Sit him on your lap and talk to him quietly to gain his confidence (3). Make the dose as small as possible by not adding too much water, if any (3). Give it in a coloured or patterned cup or glass if one is available (1). Show him the sweet you have for him after he has taken his 'drink' (3). He may like to drink it through a straw (3).

If he refuses, try telling him a story (3); show him the bottle with his own name on it (2); show him the other children taking their medicines (3). Tell him it will make him better so he can soon go home (3). When he has taken the dose, tell him what a good, brave boy he is (3). His mother may be able to give it him without any fuss (3) and may know a game he likes to play while he is drinking it (3).

(b) *How you would help a child to settle on his first night in hospital* (34 marks)

His mother (*or* father) should be allowed to do as much as possible for the child and to make it as much like they do at home: give him a wash or bath (2), give him his usual supper (2), clean his teeth (2), read him a story (2) and tuck him up with a favourite toy (2). The mother can stay until he is asleep (2). (If the mother cannot stay, the nurse must do the above.)

The nurse should find out whether the child usually sleeps with a light on or off, and can try and make a similar condition in the ward (5).

She should also ask if he is woken up for toilet purposes, if he is dry at night or still wears a napkin (10).

Try not to wake the child up once he is asleep (4). If he should wake, go to him at once in case he is frightened; reassure him by staying until he is asleep again (3).

(c) *How you would care for a child who has just vomited* (33 marks)

Comfort the child (5) and explain that he was sick because he is not well and that he will soon be better (3).

Without fuss, take the child to the bathroom, if possible, to wash and change him *or* wash the child in bed and change his nightclothes (6 for either). Help him clean his teeth and use a mouthwash (4).

Change the bedlinen as necessary (2). Put a vomit bowl and cloth on his locker so he can reach them if he feels sick again (3).

Let him rest on or in his bed (2) and explain why he should not eat or drink for a while (2).

Report to sister the time he vomited (2), the amount (2) and the nature of the vomit (*or* whether it occurred after a meal or medicine) (2).

Paediatric Nursing

14 INFANTILE DIARRHOEA AND VOMITING

REVISION QUIZ

In each of questions 1–8 there is only ONE correct answer. You have to choose this; so write A, B or C, etc., ONLY.

1. A baby with diarrhoea and vomiting has been put on intravenous fluids. Is this mainly necessary

   A. to supply him with nourishment
   B. to prevent dehydration
   C. to prevent anaemia
   D. to raise his blood pressure

2. Which one of the following methods might also be used for a baby with diarrhoea and vomiting

   A. subcutaneous infusion B. oesophageal feeding
   C. rectal infusion

3. Is diarrhoea and vomiting more likely to occur

   A. in a breast-fed baby B. in a bottle-fed baby

4. When the baby has stopped vomiting, which of the following is most likely to be given first by mouth

   A. diluted cow's milk
   B. diluted breast milk
   C. breast milk
   D. half-strength normal saline and glucose

5. Should a baby with diarrhoea and vomiting be nursed

   A. in a separate room or cubicle
   B. behind screens in a corner of the main ward
   C. in either one or the other

6. Which of the following additional duties would be the safest for a nurse who was looking after a baby with diarrhoea and vomiting to carry out

A. making up feeds
B. serving meals to older children
C. bathing older children
D. bathing other babies

7. Which of the following is the correct procedure before a nurse attends to the baby

A. wash hands, put on gloves, then gown
B. put on gown, wash hands, then gloves
C. wash hands, put on gown, wash hands, then gloves.
D. put on mask, then gloves, then gown

8. Which of the following is correct after the nurse has finished

A. discard gloves; wash and dry hands; remove gown
B. remove gown; discard gloves; wash and dry hands
C. discard gloves; remove gown; wash and dry hands

Now WRITE answers to the following questions.

9. List any special charts and records which should be kept when nursing a baby with diarrhoea and vomiting.

10. List any disposable articles which could be used in nursing this baby.

11. List instructions you should give to the mother if she is helping with the baby.

12. List any steps the nursing staff looking after other babies and children should take to protect them from infection with the diarrhoea and vomiting.

Now correct your answers from the notes on pages 107 and 108.

ANSWERS AND NOTES ON REVISION QUIZ

For questions 1–8 count TWO marks for each correct answer.

Correct answer

1. B. Babies with diarrhoea or diarrhoea and vomiting very quickly become dehydrated, and can die from this.

2. A. Subcutaneous infusion may be used. Oesophageal feeding cannot be used while the baby is vomiting; it may be necessary later if he is too weak to suck.

3. B. Bottle-fed babies are more liable to diarrhoea and vomiting. So if the baby has been breast-fed, he will be put back on the breast as soon as he can keep feeds down.

4. D. Feeding has to be started very carefully. Probably half-strength normal saline and glucose at first; if this stays down, diluted cows' or breast milk; then on to normal feeding—all taking 3 to 5 days. In a young bottle-fed baby skimmed or half-cream artificial milk may be given until his usual feed can be resumed, in preference to giving diluted cows' milk.

5. A. As this is very infectious among babies, and all the ways in which it spreads are not known, he should be in a separate room or cubicle, with the door *kept shut*.

6. C. Older children are not nearly so likely to catch this infection; so bathing them should be safe. But the nurse should not go into the kitchen or milk kitchen or touch the children's food.

7. C. Wash hands, put on gown, wash hands, then gloves. After washing, the *gown* is put on before the nurse has touched anything inside the cubicle, so that her hands, which are socially clean, do not infect the inside of the sleeves, which touch her clothes. After washing again, disposable *gloves* are then put on to keep her hands from becoming infected.

8. A. Discard gloves, wash and dry hands and remove gown. *Gloves* are heavily contaminated; they must not be worn when removing the gown, as they will infect the inside of the sleeves. They are discarded first into a paper sack. *Hands* are then washed, as they may have become contaminated when removing the gloves. Finally the *gown* is removed, care being taken only to handle its 'clean' inside, and hung up. Hands are washed again outside the cubicle.

For questions 9–12 count marks as shown.

9. Amount of fluid intake (2), intravenous or subcutaneous (1), by oesophageal tube (1) or by mouth (1); and types of fluid taken (2). Record of each stool passed (2) and its character (2) (i.e. whether green, normal colour, liquid or partly formed). Record of each time of vomiting (2).

10. Napkins (2), gloves (2) and paper towels (2) are the most important items. Equipment such as gallipots, oesophageal tube, syringe barrel, sheets (1 mark for any one).

11. Instructions as to gown (1), gloves (1) and handwashing (1) (as above); not to go into the kitchen (1) or touch other babies (1).

12. Other staff must not enter infected child's cubicle (2); must watch for diarrhoea in other children so that they can be isolated immediately (2); must see that all children's hands are washed after going to lavatory (2) and before meals (2); must report if she herself has diarrhoea and go off duty (2).

Maximum Total = 51 marks.

Your score will show you how well you have done. Do any more revision which you think you need BEFORE attempting the question on the page opposite.

QUESTION

Without looking back, or consulting any book, write the answer to the question on this page. You should not take more than 40 minutes to plan and write your answer.

A baby in the paediatric unit develops diarrhoea and vomiting.

(a) What nursing care will this baby require?
(b) What measures will be taken to prevent this infection spreading to other children in the unit?

When you have finished your answer, and not before, turn over and correct it by the 'model answer' overleaf.

MODEL ANSWER

(a) *Nursing care* (50 marks)

Babies with diarrhoea and vomiting quickly become dehydrated (2), so this baby will probably be given fluids intravenously or subcutaneously until vomiting stops (2). The nurse must make sure that the fluid is running in at the required rate (2) and no faster (2), and that the needle is still in position (2).

When he has stopped vomiting, the baby will have to be bottle-fed (1), probably with half-strength normal saline with glucose (2). This must be done slowly (2), making sure he does not swallow too much air (2). Small quantities are given at first and increased if he keeps them down (2).

If he is too weak to suck, he may be fed by a small oesophageal tube (2). This is lubricated (1), and passed into the stomach (1). The nurse should make quite sure that the tube is in the stomach, usually by aspirating a small amount of stomach contents (1). The feed is then poured down the barrel of a syringe attached to the tube (1).

As his condition improves, he will be fed with diluted cows' milk or breast milk (2); and over the next two or three days get back to normal bottle feeds (2) or to breast-feeding (2).

All fluids taken by any route must be measured and recorded (2).

The baby should be handled very gently (3). When his napkins are changed his buttocks should be carefully washed (1) and dried (1) and barrier cream (*or* examples such as Thovaline, zinc and castor oil ointment) applied to prevent them becoming sore (2).

The baby's mother should be allowed to help in his care as far as she is able (5).

A chart must be kept recording each stool passed (2) and its character (1), and any vomiting recorded (2).

(b) *Measures to prevent spread of infection* (50 marks)

The baby must be isolated in a separate room or cubicle (2) and the door kept shut (2). The nurses who look after him must not make up feeds (2) or attend to other babies (3). If the infection is serious, no other babies under one year should be admitted (2), and those in the unit should be sent home as soon as possible (*or* transferred as soon as possible) (2).

Anything taken into the cubicle must be disinfected at once when it is taken out (2). Linen is put into a dissolvable plastic bag or soaked in antiseptic before being sent to the laundry (2). Disposable articles such as napkins are used if possible (2). These are put into a paper sack (2) before being removed to be incinerated (2).

Before attending to the baby, the nurse puts on gown (3) and disposable gloves (3). After finishing, she removes gloves (3), washes her hands (3), removes the gown (2) and washes her hands again (2). The mother must also take these precautions (3).

Any other child developing diarrhoea should be isolated and the same precautions taken (2). Any member of staff with diarrhoea must be sent off duty (2).

Staff in the unit must see that all the children's hands are always washed after going to the lavatory (2) and before meals (2).

Paediatric Nursing

15 EPILEPSY

REVISION QUIZ

In questions 1–3 there is only ONE correct answer. You have to choose this; so write A, B or C, etc., ONLY.

1. A known epileptic often has a warning (or aura) of an impending attack. Is the aura most likely to take the form of

   A. twitching of all the limbs
   B. cessation of pulse and respirations
   C. mental confusion
   D. crying out
   E. sudden unconsciousness

2. A patient has an epileptic fit when up in the ward. Would you *first*

   A. send for a doctor
   B. go and fetch sister
   C. put the patient to bed
   D. sit him on a chair
   E. lay him flat on the floor

3. In the convulsive stage of the attack, which is the most essential

   A. to keep the patient quiet
   B. to prevent him hurting himself
   C. to give him a drink
   D. to restrain him forcefully

Now WRITE answers to the following questions.

4. List the articles which should be found by the bed of an epileptic patient.

5. List the things you would report to sister, or doctor, after a patient has had an epileptic fit.

Now correct your answers from the notes on page 114.

ANSWERS AND NOTES ON REVISION QUIZ

For questions 1–3 count TWO marks for each correct answer.

Correct answer

1. D. Some patients have other kinds of warning: hear noises, smell specific odours, taste curious tastes, etc. Crying out is the commonest, especially with children.

2. E. The attack is likely to come on very soon after the aura: this is the quickest thing to do with safety.

3. B. He may bruise himself by knocking into furniture; he may be holding someting on which he could cut himself; he may be near a fire or heater; he may bite his tongue.

For questions 4 and 5 count marks as shown.

4. None. Modern management follows a policy of non-intervention to avoid oral, dental or respiratory trauma. Count TWO marks.

5. time the attack started
   whether or not there was an aura
   type of aura
   time between aura and convulsions
   time convulsions lasted
   where convulsions started (or whether eyes, arms, legs twitched first)
   whether he became blue or stopped breathing
   whether or not he was incontinent
   whether he hurt himself (or bit his tongue)
   if he became unconscious
   his present state
   his temperature, pulse and respiration rate

Count ONE mark for each point mentioned: *possible total* = 12 marks.

Maximum Total = 20 marks.

Your score will show you how well you have done. Do any more revision which you think you need BEFORE attempting the question on the page opposite.

QUESTION

Without looking back or consulting any book, write the answer to the question on this page. You should not take more than 40 minutes to plan and write your answer.

A child in the ward has an epileptic fit.

(a) What first aid treatment would you carry out?
(b) What observations would you make and report on this child during the fit?

When you have finished your answer, and not before, turn over and correct it by the 'model answer' overleaf.

MODEL ANSWER

(a) *First aid treatment* (50 marks)

Go to the child at once (5) and remove any toy, cup, glass or nearby furniture (10 for any TWO examples) so he does not hurt himself (2).

If the child shows signs of asphyxia during the convulsion, he should be turned to the 'coma' position to maintain a clear airway. The nurse should remain with the child, not restraining him, while the fit lasts (10).

During the convulsions, the child's head should be turned to one side to prevent inhalation of saliva (*or* to allow saliva to drain out of his mouth) (8).

Another person should inform sister (3) and can fetch a blanket to cover the patient (2). She can also keep other children away, or put a screen round so they will not be frightened (3).

As soon as possible (*or* after the convulsions) the child is lifted on to his bed and allowed to sleep (4).

The child should be reassured, and also his parents if they are there, throughout the attack (3).

(b) *Observations you would make and report during the fit* (50 marks)

The time at which the attack started (2).

Whether or not there was a warning (*or* aura) (5) and the form this took (*or* whether the child cried out) (2).

The length of time betwee the aura and the start of the convulsions (2).

Were there eye movements during the convulsive stage and did these occur before or after other movements? (3). Which limbs started 'twitching' first (2). The length of time of this stage (2).

Whether or not the child was incontinent during the fit (3).

The nurse should find out whether the child hurt himself (4) or bit his tongue (4). She should report if he became cyanosed (*or* blue) (3) or held his breath and for how long (2).

After the actual fit, whether the child became unconscious and for how long (4).

The nurse should report on his present condition: whether sleeping, awake, fretful or quiet (4 for any TWO suggestions).

His temperature, pulse and respirations should have been taken after the attack and abnormalities reported (4).

The child may not remember anything about the fit—this too should be reported (2). His parents' presence or absence should be mentioned as they would need to to be told when they next visited (2).

Paediatric Nursing

16 BLOOD: CARE OF CHILD HAVING BLOOD TRANSFUSION

REVISION QUIZ

In each of questions 1–9, there is only ONE correct answer. You have to choose this; so write A, B or C, etc., ONLY.

1. Which of the following describes the composition of blood plasma
   A. water, mineral salts and blood cells
   B. blood proteins, mineral salts and water
   C. food substances, water and haemoglobin
   D. water, food substances and oxygen

2. The number of red cells in 1 mm^3 (cubic millimetre) of blood is approximately

A. 50 000 000	B. 5000 000	C. 100 000
D. 50 000	E. 10 000	F. 1000

3. The number of white cells in 1 mm^3 (cubic millimetre) of blood is approximately

A. 50 000 000	B. 5000 000	C. 100 000
D. 50 000	E. 10 000	F. 1000

4. Is the function of red blood cells to carry
   A. oxygen
   B. oxygen and carbon dioxide
   C. oxygen and food
   D. oxygen, carbon dioxide and food

5. One kind of white blood cell is the *polymorph* (or polymorphonuclear cell). Do polymorphs
   A. produce antibodies
   B. help in the clotting of blood
   C. transport food substances
   D. engulf (or ingest) bacteria

6. The other main kind of white cell is the *lymphocyte*. Does this
   A. produce antibodies
   B. help in the clotting of blood
   C. transport food substances
   D. engulf (or ingest) bacteria

7. Do the blood platelets (thrombocytes)

   A. produce antibodies
   B. help in the clotting of blood
   C. transport food substances
   D. engulf (or ingest) bacteria

8. The diagrams below represent three different kinds of blood cell. Which is correct

A. I = red cell	II = polymorph	III = lymphocyte
B. I = polymorph	II = red cell	III = lymphocyte
C. I = lymphocyte	II = polymorph	III = red cell
D. I = red cell	II = lymphocyte	III = polymorph

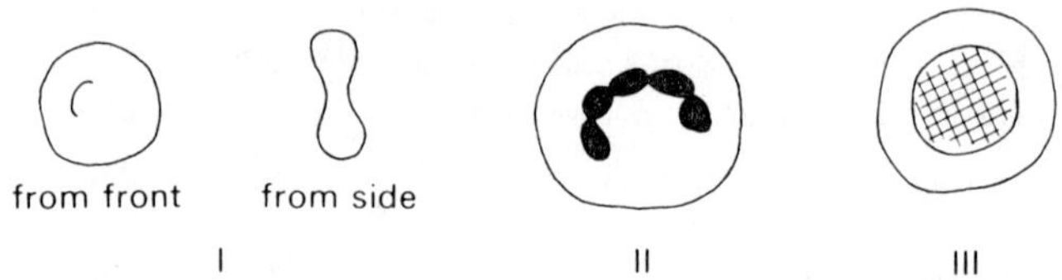

9. When a bottle of blood has to be given in a transfusion, who should check it? Is it

   A. the sister or nurse in charge of the ward
   B. two nurses
   C. a nurse and a doctor
   D. the sister and a doctor

Now WRITE answers to the following questions.

10. List the details which you would find on

   (a) the label of a bottle of blood
   (b) the form from the laboratory which must be used in checking the blood

11. Briefly state what you mean by 'cross-matching' blood.

12. A child is having a blood transfusion. List

   (a) ways in which he can be kept happy
   (b) the nursing care he requires
   (c) the care required to the apparatus
   (d) observations you would make

Now correct your answers from the notes on pages 119–21.

ANSWERS AND NOTES ON REVISION QUIZ

For questions 1–9, count TWO marks for each correct answer.

Correct answer

1. B. Plasma is the fluid part of blood which transports substances to and from the body's cells. It is mainly water. It is sticky because of the proteins it contains and salty because of the mineral salts. It does contain food substances, but answer 'C' is wrong as only red cells contain haemoglobin. Red cells also carry the oxygen, so answer 'D' is also wrong.

2. B.
3. E.

(2 and 3) Perhaps it would help you to remember that there are 500 red cells to every 1 white cell.

4. A. This is their *only* function.

5. D. These are the cells that move about like an amoeba; they 'eat' like an amoeba, by engulfing food particles and germs.

6. A. White cells are therefore 'fighters of infection', but both kinds perform this function in a different way.

7. B. These increase in number when there is a wound to form a *clot*.

8. A. Diagram I = disc-shaped red cell
Diagram II = polymorph, a cell with a many-shaped nucleus
Diagram III = lymphocyte with a large round nucleus

9. B. This is the *best* choice. TWO people *must* check it as mistakes are less likely to occur. A doctor may be there at the time. You can count ONE mark if you chose answer C or D, but NONE if you chose answer A.

10. (a) The full name of the patient
His hospital number
The name or number of the ward
The blood group
The Rhesus positive/Rhesus negative information (Rh +ve/Rh −ve)
The expiry date
The serial number of the bottle.

(b) The same as above omitting the expiry date. In some hospitals the patient's age is included.

Count ONE mark for each point.

Total = 14 marks.

11. A sample of the patient's blood (1) is mixed with a sample of blood from the bottle (1). If the blood is seen to form tiny clumps (2) it is not compatible (or the wrong group) (1).

12. (a) By being allowed to have a toy or other object to which he is attached in bed with him
Letting his mother stay with him, read to him, tell him a story (1 for any ONE suggestion)
If old enough, letting him read or watch television
Explain why the transfusion is needed and what the doctor is doing and when he will feel the 'prick'
Praise him for good behaviour and for being brave

(b) Making sure he is comfortable in bed
Supporting his arm (or leg) on a pillow
Attaching it to a splint to prevent sudden movement dislodging the needle
Helping him with drinks and food
Offering him urinals or bedpans at intervals
Washing his face and hands as necessary

(c) Making sure the blood is running at the rate required
Making sure the tubing is not kinked
Observing the needle area to make sure it is not dislodged or becoming bruised or swollen and painful
When the bottle is nearly finished, ask what is to follow or if the apparatus is to be taken down

(d) Maintain a fluid balance chart
Record his temperature and pulse every hour
Observe for skin rashes
Report any loin pain at once
Report any symptoms such as nausea, vomiting, convulsions or blood in the urine

For this question, count ONE mark for each point mentioned.

Total=20 marks.

Maximum Total=57 marks.

Your score will show you how well you have done. Do any more revision which you think you need BEFORE attempting the question on page 123.

QUESTION

Without looking back or consulting any book, write the answer to the question on this page. You should not take more than 40 minutes to plan and write your answer.

A child needs a blood transfusion.

(a) Give a short description of the blood.
(b) What precautions are taken to ensure the correct blood is given?
(c) How would you manage the child during the transfusion?

When you have finished your answer, and not before, turn over and correct it by the 'model answer' overleaf.

MODEL ANSWER

(a) *Composition of blood* (40 marks)

Blood consists of a fluid part (1) called plasma (2) and blood cells (2).

Plasma is straw-coloured (1) and contains water (2), mineral salts (2), proteins (2), dissolved food substances (2) and waste materials (*or* urea and carbon dioxide) (2).

Cells: Red cells (*or* erythrocytes) (2) carry oxygen (2) (N.B. If you have said they carry *food* and oxygen, count *no* marks). They pick up oxygen as blood passes through the lungs (2) and are able to do so because they contain haemoglobin (2). They are very minute, flat discs (1) and are dark in colour because of the haemoglobin (1).

White cells (*or* leucocytes) (2) help defend the body against bacteria (*or* germs, *or* infections) (2). They are larger than red cells (1) and fewer in number (1).

There are two main types: Lymphocytes (1) which carry antibodies (1) and polymorphonuclear cells (*or* polymorphs.) (1) which engulf bacteria (1). Both types increase in number in infections (1).

Platelets (1) are small and irregular in shape and help in clotting (2).

(b) *Precautions* (15 marks)

A sample of the child's blood is taken (1) to enable it to be grouped (1) and cross-matched (1) to a bottle of blood (*or* donor blood) (1). The Rhesus factor is also ascertained (1) as Rhesus-positive blood must not be given to a Rhesus-negative child (2).

If no reactions occur when the bloods are mixed, it will be safe to use (*or* the blood will be compatible) (1).

When a bottle of blood is put up or changed, it must be carefully checked (2) against the laboratory form and the serial number on the bottle (2). This is done by two people (1).

The expiry date on the bottle of blood should be checked to make sure it is fresh enough to be used (2).

(c) *Management of the child during transfusion* (45 marks)

If old enough the child should be told a little about the transfusion (1) and that he will feel a little prick in his arm (1). He will be asked to keep very still to help the doctor (1). He can also be told that the blood will make him feel better and he will soon be able to go home (2).

His mother, or a nurse, should hold his hand and read him a story while the transfusion is being put up (3) and while it is in progress (1). It will help if he can have a favourite toy or other object to which he is attached in bed with him (1).

The limb used should be lightly splinted (1) and rested on a protected pillow (1). He should be made comfortable in bed (1) and helped with drinks and food as allowed (1).

His mother, or the nurse sitting with him, should keep a close watch on the transfusion to see it is kept running at the required rate (3) and to call for help if it stops (2).

The child's temperature and pulse should be taken and recorded every hour (3) and any rise reported at once (2). Other signs of transfusion reaction should also be observed: rigors, convulsions, pain in the loin, nausea, vomiting or skin rashes (4 for any FOUR mentioned).

Should the child fall asleep, the mother or nurse should keep him under close observation in case he suddenly wakes or moves in his sleep and disturbs the transfusion (3).

A fluid balance chart should be kept (3) and the blood recorded as 'intake' when it has run through (1).

The mother can wash his hands and face (2), give him a urinal or 'potty' (2), and help the nurse make his bed (2) as this will keep the child happy and also help to allay his mother's anxiety (2).

If any reactions occur, help should be summoned at once as the transfusion may have to be stopped (2).

Paediatric Nursing

17 CEREBRAL PALSY

REVISION QUIZ

1. A child with cerebral palsy (a 'spastic') is being admitted to your ward. List the points you would enter on his notes about his personal 'data'.

2. What would you want to ask his mother about

   (a) his eating habits
   (b) his toilet habits
   (c) his daily routine

3. List some of the problems you may encounter with a spastic child in a busy children's ward.

4. What help may be available for this child in the community

   (a) for his home
   (b) towards his training
   (c) for his mother

5. List the steps you would take to help this child settle into the ward.

6. List any suitable ways you can think of for occupying this child's time while he is in hospital.

Now correct your answers from the notes on pages 128 and 129.

ANSWERS AND NOTES ON REVISION QUIZ

Count marks as indicated.

1. Full name (1)
   Date of birth and age (1)
   Home address (1)
   Parents' address if different from home address (1)
   Telephone number (1)
   Name and address of general practitioner (1)
   Religion (1)
   Whether baptized or not (1)
   Infectious diseases had (1)
   Immunizations (1)
   Whether he is having any medicines (1)
   Any allergies (1)

2. (a) Which foods he likes or dislikes (2)
   How much help he needs at mealtimes? (*or* can he feed himself?) (2)
   Is he able to chew food properly? (2)
   (b) Is he continent of urine and faeces? (1)
   Is he dry at night? (1)
   Is he able to ask when he requires toilet facilities? (1)
   Are his bowels regular? (1)
   Which laxatives are given when needed? (1)
   Does he wear protective clothing or napkins? (1)
   (c) Does he sleep restfully and for how long? (2)
   What time does he get up? (1)
   What time does he go to bed? (1)
   How does he spend his day? (1)
   What does he like to do? (*or* does he like radio, television, reading, being read to, playing with other children?) (2)

3. Difficulties with communicating for other children, staff–child may not be able to speak or may not speak distinctly (2)
   He may fall (if walking), or injure himself on unfamiliar furniture, toys or equipment (2)
   Much patience and time may be needed at mealtimes, in dealing with his toilet requirements and in gaining his confidence (2)
   Other children may be frightened if he is unable to speak and if his appearance is affected very much (2)
   Excessive salivation may be a problem and he may need to wear a bib or have frequent changes of clothing (2)
   In strange surroundings his spasticity may increase for a time (2)

4. (a) Fitting of hand-rails so the child can be encouraged to walk (1)
If he is confined to a wheelchair, ramps may be needed for the doorsteps (1)
Window-bars may be needed if child very active (1)
Stairs should be fitted with a gate to prevent falls (1)
A wheelchair would be provided and a larger one obtained as the child grows (2)

(b) Physiotherapy to help the child relax, walk and gain some degree of independence (2)
Speech therapy (2)
Nursery school, play centre or special school for the physically (and/or mentally) handicapped child (2)
Provision of hearing aid and/or spectacles as required (2)

(c) Child-minding facilities to enable her to get out at regular intervals (1)
A home teacher if child unable to go to school or centre (1)
Arrangements for child to be admitted to hospital while parents have an annual holiday (2)
Regular visiting by health visitor to give advice and support (1)

5. If possible one nurse should spend time gaining the child's confidence and doing as much as she can for him (3)
Try to keep to his home routine as much as possible (2)
Let his mother stay until he is settled (2)
Encourage another child to talk and play with him (2)
Show him the other children and the toys (2)
Let him watch television if he does this at home (2)
Avoid his becoming cross as this may lead to temper tantrums (2)

6. Suitable toys, books, drawing paper and crayons (2)
Radio (1)
Television (1)
Out in garden if fine (2)
'Play lady' or ward teacher (2)
Staff should give time to talk and play with child—he may not be used to other children (2)

Maximum Total=87 marks.

Your score will show you how well you have done. Do any more revision you think you need BEFORE attempting the question on page 131.

QUESTION

Without looking back or consulting any book, write the answer to the question on this page. You should not take more than 40 minutes to plan and write your answer.

A five-year-old spastic child is admitted to the ward for two weeks to allow the mother to have a holiday.

(a) What information is required from the mother?
(b) How can the nurse help with the special problems that arise in caring for a spastic child?
(c) List some of the organizations in the community to help the handicapped child and his family.

When you have finished your answer, and not before, turn over and correct it by the 'model answer' overleaf.

MODEL ANSWER

TO THE STUDENT. The fact that this child is to be admitted to allow his parents to have a holiday (without him) implies that this child is severely handicapped physically. He may, or may not, be mentally handicapped also.

For easy marking, part (a) of this answer has been divided into three parts, each carrying a possible 10 marks.

(a) *Information required from the mother* (30 marks)

Personal particulars: Full name (1); home address (1); parents' holiday address (1); telephone number (holiday) (1); age and date of birth (1); religion (1); whether baptized (1); name and address of general practitioner (1); immunization and vaccination particulars (1); infectious diseases (1).

How much can the child do? Can he walk unaided, with a frame or with help (1)? Can he wash or dress himself at all (1)? Can he talk (*or* make himself understood by strangers) (1)? Can he understand other people (1)? Can he hear and see normally (1)? Does he sit well in a chair, wheelchair or does he need reins to prevent falls (2)?

Does he ask for drinks, toilet facilities (1)?

Does he play or look at books (1) or watch television (1)?

His daily routine: What time does he wake up and get up (1)? What foods does he like or dislike and is able to chew (2)? Are his bowels regular or does he need aperients (1)? Is he taking any form of medicine, if so can the mother give details (*or* has she brought it with her) (2)? What time does he go to bed (1)? Does he sleep in a bed or cot (1)? Is he continent or incontinent (1) or does he need napkins (1)?

(b) *Special problems* (40 marks)

Nurses should try to gain the child's confidence (1) by talking to him (1) and spending time playing with him (1). She should try to treat him as a normal child (2); it may help to get another child to play with him (2).

If he can be happily occupied it will help to prevent homesickness (3).

The child should be kept calm as spastic children are prone to temper tantrums and this can be very upsetting to the other children (2).

At mealtimes he may need feeding (1) or his food cut up for him (1); he will probably need a bib (1). Excessive salivation (*or* dribbling) may be a problem and his clothes may need protection all the time (2).

He will need regular toilet training (2); if incontinent he must be changed immediately and his skin kept clean and dry (2). This should be done with as little fuss as possible and away from the other children (2).

His bed will need protection with waterproof sheets (2) and cot-sides may also be needed as these children are often restless (2).

It may be his first time away from his mother and he will need constant reassurance that she will be back in '*x*' days time (3).

Nurses must see that he eats and drinks enough as he may be unwilling to do so at first (2). If he can be taken into the garden during the day, this will help keep him well (2).

'Play lady' or teacher may be able to keep him amused and he should be helped to take part in the ward activities as much as possible (3).

Great care must be taken to see he does not injure himself by falling or rough treatment by bigger children (3).

(c) *Help available in the community* (30 marks)

School for physically handicapped children (3)
Play centres or home teachers in special cases (4)
Spastic Society (a voluntary organization) (2)
Health Visitor to give advice (2)
Laundry services in cases of incontinence (2)
Home Help service to allow mother to go out shopping or to have a little recreation (3)
Red Cross may lend nursing aids, wheelchair or walking frame (4)
Local Authority may allow money for alterations to the home, e.g. rails along walls to help child walk; stair-rails; window bars; safety gate for top of stairs; ramp for wheelchair if child very heavy (4 for any 2 suggestions)
General practitioner (2)
Child psychologist to assess mental ability (2)
Physiotherapist to teach child to relax and become less spastic (2)

Paediatric Nursing

18 TREATMENT FOR HEAD LICE

REVISION QUIZ

WRITE answers to the following questions.

1. List the articles you would need to disinfest the head of a child with head lice.

2. List the measures you would take to prevent the lice spreading to

   (a) yourself
   (b) other patients in the ward

In questions 3–6 there is only ONE correct answer. You have to choose this; so write A, B or C, etc., ONLY.

3. In treating the head of a child, who has long hair, with lice, would you

   A. first cut her hair short
   B. treat it then cut her hair short
   C. leave her hair long

4. Would you

   A. apply lotion to the hair, then fine-comb it
   B. fine-comb the hair and then apply lotion

5. Having treated the hair would you

   A. cover it with a cap
   B. put on a capelline bandage
   C. leave it uncovered

6. After first treating the hair, how soon will the child be completely free of lice and nits

   A. immediately B. next day C. after 3 days
   D. after 8 days E. after a month

Now correct your answers from the notes on page 136.

ANSWERS AND NOTES ON REVISION QUIZ

For questions 1 and 2 count marks as shown.

1. A shoulder cape (for the child) (1)
   Brush and comb (1)
   A steel nit comb (*or* Sacker's comb) (1)
   Squares of old linen (*or* swabs) (1)
   A gallipot of antiseptic (1)
   Disposal bag for used swabs (1)
   Lotion: lethane oil *or* DDT *or* Lorexane 1:4 (1)
   For the nurse: a triangular bandage for her head (1)
   a gown (1)
   Total=9 marks.

2. (a) Cover your own hair completely before starting (2).
   Wear a gown which should be sent to the laundry afterwards (2).
   (b) Keep the infested child's brush, comb, towels and clothing separately (2).
   When treatment is complete, change all the child's bedlinen and nightclothes (2).
   Observe the other children for signs of lice (*or* for scratching *or* nits) (2).

In the following questions, count TWO marks for each correct answer.

Correct answer

3. C. There is no need to cut it. In any case, a child's hair should *never* be cut without written consent from the parent.
4. B. You should remove as many lice and nits as possible first. This may take a long time if heavily infested.

5. C. With modern lotions it is not necessary to make the child conspicuous by covering her hair.

6. D. Lice take 8 days to hatch out from the nits (eggs). The lotion will kill them as they hatch out.

Maximum Total=27 marks.

Your score will show you how well you have done. Do any more revision which you think you need BEFORE attempting the question on the page opposite.

QUESTION

Without looking back or consulting any book, write the answer to the question on this page. You should not take more than 40 minutes to plan and write your answer.

A small girl is admitted to your ward and is found to have head lice. She is frightened and neglected.

(a) How will you handle the child?
(b) What measures will you take to prevent the lice spreading to other patients and yourself?

When you have finished your answer, and not before, turn over and correct it by the 'model answer' overleaf.

MODEL ANSWER

(a) *Handling the child* (80 marks)

Nurse must not attach any blame to the child and be kind and gentle towards her (4). Other children should not be told (2) and the patient should not be kept away from them (2). Treatment should be done in the clinical room (*or* out of sight of other children) (1).

The child should be constantly reassured that treatment does not hurt (1), that she will soon be better (1) and she will be able to go home (1) and back to school (1). She should also be told that her parents and brothers and sisters will come to see here (2) and maybe bring her presents (1). She should be shown the ward's toys (2) and any other children of her age (2). Radio and television will also help to amuse her (2).

If possible the child should be given pretty clothes (2) and articles for washing as she probably did not come in supplied with these (2). She must be encouraged to look 'smart' and praised when she washes herself or cleans her teeth (2).

The nurse can gain the child's confidence by explaining any treatment (2).

To treat the hair a tray is set containing:

a shoulder cape (1)
brush and comb (1)
a steel nit comb (*or* Sacker's comb) (2)
squares of old linen or swabs (1)
a gallipot of antiseptic (1)
disposal bag for used swabs (1)
DDT lotion (*or* lethane oil *or* Lorexane 1:4) (2 for any ONE)

The child is sat on a chair (2), her shoulders covered (2) and given a book to look at (2).

Any tangles are removed with the brush and comb (1) and the hair parted in several places (1). The lotion is dropped along the partings using a swab (*or* medicine dropper) (4). It is then rubbed in gently so that it reaches all parts of the hair (2). The hair is combed with the steel comb to remove any dead lice (4), wiping the comb each time with the linen squares which are put straight into the disposal bag (3). Particular care is taken with areas behind the ears (2).

Her hair is tidied before she goes back into the ward (2). The cape is sponged with the antiseptic and hung up to dry (3).

Each day the hair is combed with the steel comb (4) so that lice are removed as they are killed by the lotion as they hatch out from the nits (4).

On the eighth day, the hair is thoroughly examined and if free of nits (3) it can be washed and dried (2).

(b) *Preventing spread to others* (20 marks)

When attending to the child's hair, nurse should wear a gown (2) and have her own hair completely covered with a triangular bandage (4).

The patient's brush, comb, towels and clothes should be kept apart from the other children's (2).

When the hair has been washed, her brush and comb should be properly cleaned (4) and all her bedlinen and nightclothes changed (4).

During bath-time, nurses should carefully inspect the other children's heads in case they are also infested (4).

General Nursing

19 ABNORMALITIES IN URINE

REVISION QUIZ

For questions 1–4 there is only ONE correct answer. You have to choose this; so write A, B or C, etc., ONLY.

1. If acetone is found in the urine of a diabetic patient, is it likely to be due to
   A. too much insulin being given
   B. faulty fat metabolism
   C. faulty sugar metabolism
   D. too much food being taken

2. Acetone may be found in the urine of people who are not diabetics. Which of the following does *not* give rise to acetone in the urine
   A. jaundice
   B. starvation
   C. shock
   D. vomiting

3. In a diabetic patient, acetone in the urine may indicate
   A. a urinary infection
   B. pre-insulin coma
   C. pre-diabetic coma
   D. a low blood sugar

4. Why is sugar not normally found in urine? Is it because
   A. it is reabsorbed in the kidney for use by the body
   B. it is excreted by another organ
   C. it is required by the body for energy
   D. it is neutralized by insulin

5. The commonest causes for *blood* in the urine are found at the side of the chart below. The organs of the urinary system are found at the top. Place a tick in the appropriate space, to show which organs may be the cause of haematuria.

	Kidney	*Ureter*	*Bladder*	*Urethra*
Injury				
Infection				
Stones				
New growths				

Now correct your answers from the notes on page 142.

ANSWERS AND NOTES FOR REVISION QUIZ

For questions 1–4 count TWO marks for each correct answer.

Correct answer

1. B. When fats are not metabolized correctly, ketone bodies are formed: acetone is found in the urine. Due to insufficient insulin in diabetics, sugar cannot be stored and used—the body has to use fats for its supply of energy; but these are not able to be 'burnt up' normally.

2. A. All the other conditions are likely to give rise to ketonuria.

3. C. It is always a danger sign and should therefore never be ignored. Ketones are 'poisonous' to the brain and cause unconsciousness in time.

4. A. Some of you may have chosen answer 'C' which, of course is partially correct. Count ONE mark if you have done so, but it is only half the story.

5. Your chart should look like this:

	Kidney	*Ureter*	*Bladder*	*Urethra*
Injury	✓		✓	✓
Infection	✓		✓	✓
Stones	✓	✓	✓	
New growths	✓		✓	

Count ONE mark for each tick correctly placed.

Maximum Total = 17 marks.

Your score will show you how well you have done. Do any more revision you think you need BEFORE attempting the question on the page opposite.

QUESTION

Without looking back or consulting any book, write the answer to the question on this page. You should not take more than 40 minutes to plan and write your answer.

Give a short account of the significance of *any three* of the following abnormalities which may be present in urine.

(a) Blood
(b) Acetone
(c) Protein
(d) Sugar

When you have finished your answer, and not before, turn over and correct it by the 'model answer' overleaf.

MODEL ANSWER

Note to student. Remember that you should have written on only *three* of these subjects.

(a) *Blood* (33 marks)

Found following injuries to the kidney (2), bladder (1) or urethra (1), as caused by road traffic accident (*or* crushing) (1) or fractures of the lower ribs or pelvis (1). All urine should be saved so specimens can be compared for assessing whether the bleeding is stopping (2).

Tumours (*or* new growths) (2) of the kidney (1) or bladder (1) can also cause haematuria which is usually painless (2) and often not very severe (1).

Overdose of anticoagulant drugs (2) may first show itself by haematuria which is an important observation which must be reported (1).

Bleeding may also occur from the bladder or urethra after cystoscopy (1) which is often only temporary (1).

It also occurs when the prostate gland is enlarged (1) and after operations on the bladder (1) or prostate (1). If very severe it may lead to clot retention (2).

Stones anywhere in the urinary tract can cause bleeding (2) often accompanied by very severe pain (*or* renal colic) (2).

Urinary infections can cause haematuria (2) with pain on passing urine (*or* dysuria) (1); the urine may smell 'fishy' (1).

(b) *Acetone* (33 marks)

Faulty metabolism of fats may cause ketone bodies to be produced (3). usually due to diabetes (*or* lack of insulin) causing inability to use and store sugar (2). The body then has to burn its fats to produce heat and energy (3). If acetone is found in a diabetic's urine it must always be reported (2) as it may be a sign of impending coma (4). The breath will usually smell of acetone (3) and the patient may be drowsy (3). Before a diabetic patient goes home, he should be warned to inform his doctor should he find acetone in his urine (3).

Dehydration, especially in children, also causes ketonuria (3). This may be due to excessive vomiting (2); this may also occur in pregnancy (2). It is also found in shock (3).

(c) *Protein* (33 marks)

Found in any disease of the kidney (5) or urinary tract (2) such as acute glomerular nephritis (2), nephrotic syndrome (2), chronic renal failure (2). It shows that kidney cells are not filtering blood correctly (5).

It is also found in heart failure (2) and hypertension (2) due to poor blood supply to the kidneys (2).

It is sometimes found in acute infections (1). It may be a sign of early pregnancy complication (*or* pre-eclamptic toxaemia) (2).

Protein in urine is often accompanied by oedema (*or* swelling of the ankles) (3).

It also is found when there is blood in the urine, because protein is one of the constituents of blood (3).

(d) *Sugar* (33 marks)

In an otherwise stable diabetic, the presence of sugar may mean she has an acute infection (2), has diarrhoea and vomiting leading to dehydration (2), is not keeping to her diet (3) or is having the wrong dose of insulin (3). If it persists, she should go to her doctor (or it should be reported) (2).

During stabilization, the amount of sugar in the urine determines the amount of insulin the doctor orders (3), hence the importance of regular (*or* four-hourly) urine testing and accurate charts (4).

If a diabetic has no sugar in the urine, it could mean she is having too much insulin (2) and she may have a reaction (*or* insulin coma) (1).

It is safest for diabetics to have a trace of sugar in the urine (3) as long as there is no acetone (2).

In an otherwise stable diabetic, the presence of sugar may mean she has an acute infection (1), has diarrhoea and vomiting leading to dehydration (1), is not keeping to her diet (2) or is having the wrong dose of insulin (2). If it persists, she should go to her doctor (*or* it should be reported) (1).

General Nursing

20 THE CENTRAL STERILE SUPPLY DEPARTMENT

REVISION QUIZ

In each of questions 1–5 there is only ONE correct answer. You have to choose this; so write A, B or C, etc., ONLY.

1. Are spores

   A. a special kind of bacterium
   B. coverings which protect bacteria
   C. a special kind of virus
   D. kinds of fungus

2. By which of the following methods are spores efficiently destroyed

   A. boiling
   B. autoclaving
   C. baking in a hot-air oven
   D. all three of these methods
   E. either autoclaving or in a hot-air oven

3. Do articles put in an autoclave reach

   A. the boiling point of water
   B. a temperature just below this
   C. a higher temperature than this

4. Does an autoclave sterilize articles

   A. by wet heat   B. by dry heat

5. Some disposable articles of equipment come from factories. Are these sterilized

   A. by autoclave   B. in hot-air ovens   C. by gamma rays

Now WRITE answers to the following questions.

6. List some ways in which a CSSD can help to bring about economies in the Health Service.

7. What checks are made to make sure that sterilization in the CSSD is efficient?

8. What would *you* check when selecting a dressing pack to make sure that its contents were still sterile?

9. After using the dressing pack, how would you deal with

   (a) disposable articles
   (b) non-disposable articles

Now correct your answers from the notes on the next page.

ANSWERS AND NOTES ON REVISION QUIZ

For questions 1–5 count TWO marks for each correct answer.

Correct answer

1. B. Spores are waxy coverings which certain bacteria develop to protect them when they are in unfavourable surroundings—against heat, dryness, antiseptics, etc.

2. B. Autoclaving is the only reliable method of destroying spores. Bacteria which do not form spores are destroyed by heat even at temperatures below boiling point; but spore-bearing ones are much tougher. So in considering methods of sterilization, one of the main questions is 'will spores be destroyed'?

3. C. Steam under pressure in an autoclave reaches a temperature well above the normal boiling point of water. This is because the higher the pressure, the more heat is needed to cause water to boil and escape as steam.

4. A. Steam under pressure sterilizes by wet heat. The steam is then sucked out and the articles dried, so that they are dry when they leave the autoclave.

5. C. The pre-sterilized articles produced commercially are sterilized by gamma rays. These are rays which destroy living tissues, including bacteria and their spores.

For questions 6–9 count marks as shown.

6. It is more economical to buy equipment centrally than if each ward and department carried its own stock: over-ordering is avoided (2). It economizes on time: the cleaning and sterilizing is done more quickly in a department in which people do not have nursing duties as well (2). One CSSD can serve more than one hospital, and also health clinics and district nurses (2).

7. Tests are done by the pathological laboratory to make sure samples of equipment (1) and sterilizing machinery are not contaminated (1). There are also witness tubes (1) and adhesive tape on the packs (1), which change colour when they have reached the correct temperature (1).

8. You should check that there are no tears in the wrapping (1), and that the tape on the pack has changed colour (1). You should also make sure equipment is not kept too long, by using first packs which were delivered first (1).

9. (a) Disposable articles are wrapped in paper bags (1), and placed directly in the paper sack or bin provided (1).
   (b) Check instruments, etc. which have to be returned so that they do not get lost or thrown away (2). Put in the special receptacle to be returned to the CSSD (1). Nothing used is taken into clinical room where sterile equipment is kept (2).

Maximum Total = 31 marks.

Your score will show you how well you have done. Do any more revision which you think you need BEFORE attempting the question on the page opposite.

QUESTION

Without looking back or consulting any book, write the answer to the question on this page. You should not take more than 40 minutes to plan and write your answer.

(a) Describe the advantages or a Central Sterile Supply Department.
(b) What are your responsibilities when you use equipment supplied by this department?

When you have finished your answer, and not before, turn over and correct it by the 'model answer' overleaf.

MODEL ANSWER

(a) *Advantages of a Central Sterile Supply Department* (65 marks)

For several reasons, sterilization is more reliable with a Central Sterile Supply Department (5). Autoclaves (*or* steam under pressure) are one of the main ways of sterilizing, and they reach a higher temperature than if articles are boiled (5), and can destroy all spores as well as bacteria (5). Temperatures are regulated scientifically (5), and indicator tubes (2) and tape (2) show that the correct temperatures have been reached (3).

Sterility can be controlled by the pathological laboratory, which does regular tests on samples of equipment (5).

The staff of the department is entirely occupied with cleaning and sterilizing, so the work is not interfered with by other duties, as it may be on wards and departments (5).

Many articles supplied are disposable; this lessens the risk of used equipment carrying infection (5).

A CSSD ensures that the correct equipment is ready in each pack (5). It saves the time of the nursing staff (3).

Equipment is ordered centrally, which is more economical (5), and ensures that there is an adequate supply (5).

A CSSD can supply more than one hospital, and also clinics and district nurses, with reliably sterilized equipment (5).

(b) *Responsibilities in using equipment* (35 marks)

The nurse must see that packs are used in the correct order so that those supplied first are used first (*or* must not allow packs to be kept in stock for too long) (5). She must examine each pack to make sure the contents are still sterile by looking for tears in the wrapping (5) and noticing whether the indicator tape has changed colour (5). She must use non-touch technique in using equipment (5).

After use, the nurse must carefully count any instruments or equipment which has to be returned to the department, to see that nothing is lost (5). Equipment should be put straight into the correct containers to be returned (5); and nothing which has been used should be taken into the clinical room where the sterile equipment is kept (5).